This book is intended solely for informational and tracking purposes. It is not a substitute for professional medical advice, diagnosis, or treatment. Always consult a qualified healthcare provider regarding any medical concerns, symptoms, questions, and/or conditions. The publisher, author, and associated contractors assume no responsibility for any decisions made based on the information contained within this book. If you have a medical emergency, seek immediate assistance from a licensed medical professional.

Published by House of Sanchez LLC
HOUSEOFSANCHEZ.COM

MEDICAL PROVIDER LIST

NAME:

SPECIALTY:

PHONE:

EMAIL:

WEBSITE:

NEXT APPOINTMENT:

NOTES:

NAME:

SPECIALTY:

PHONE:

EMAIL:

WEBSITE:

NEXT APPOINTMENT:

NOTES:

NAME:

SPECIALTY:

PHONE:

EMAIL:

WEBSITE:

NEXT APPOINTMENT:

NOTES:

NAME:

SPECIALTY:

PHONE:

EMAIL:

WEBSITE:

NEXT APPOINTMENT:

NOTES:

MEDICAL PROVIDER LIST

NAME:

SPECIALTY:

PHONE:

EMAIL:

WEBSITE:

NEXT APPOINTMENT:

NOTES:

NAME:

SPECIALTY:

PHONE:

EMAIL:

WEBSITE:

NEXT APPOINTMENT:

NOTES:

NAME:

SPECIALTY:

PHONE:

EMAIL:

WEBSITE:

NEXT APPOINTMENT:

NOTES:

NAME:

SPECIALTY:

PHONE:

EMAIL:

WEBSITE:

NEXT APPOINTMENT:

NOTES:

MEDICATION LIST

MEDICINE NAME:

DOSAGE:

UNITS:

PHARMACY:

PRESCRIPTION #:

NEXT REFILL DATE:

NOTES:

MEDICINE NAME:

DOSAGE:

UNITS:

PHARMACY:

PRESCRIPTION #:

NEXT REFILL DATE:

NOTES:

MEDICINE NAME:

DOSAGE:

UNITS:

PHARMACY:

PRESCRIPTION #:

NEXT REFILL DATE:

NOTES:

MEDICINE NAME:

DOSAGE:

UNITS:

PHARMACY:

PRESCRIPTION #:

NEXT REFILL DATE:

NOTES:

MEDICATION LIST

MEDICINE NAME:

DOSAGE:

UNITS:

PHARMACY:

PRESCRIPTION #:

NEXT REFILL DATE:

NOTES:

MEDICINE NAME:

DOSAGE:

UNITS:

PHARMACY:

PRESCRIPTION #:

NEXT REFILL DATE:

NOTES:

MEDICINE NAME:

DOSAGE:

UNITS:

PHARMACY:

PRESCRIPTION #:

NEXT REFILL DATE:

NOTES:

MEDICINE NAME:

DOSAGE:

UNITS:

PHARMACY:

PRESCRIPTION #:

NEXT REFILL DATE:

NOTES:

INSTRUCTIONS

Fill out each page using the dosage and instructions given to you by your medical provider. Consult your medical provider with any questions regarding your care.

Please note: Any dosage or calculations used in this journal are for example purposes only. Consult your medical provider about specific dosages and calculations.

DEFINITIONS

BS - Blood Sugar (*from CGM or finger blood stick*)

Units - Insulin dosage units

Target Blood Sugar - The blood sugar goal received from the medical provider

Carbohydrate (Carb) Ratio - The total grams of carbohydrates per one unit of insulin received from the medical provider. *For example: 1 unit of insulin = 16 grams of carbs*

Correction Factor - This number is received from the medical provider.

Correction Dose - The amount of insulin needed to correct the blood sugar above the target blood sugar. To calculate this amount, use the following as an example:

Blood Sugar (BS) = 154
Target Blood Sugar (TBS) = 120
Correction Factor (CF) = 60

Correction Dose = (BS - TBS)/CF
= (154-120)/60
= 34/60
= **0.57 units of insulin**

Carb Dose Calculation -
Total carb amount for the meal divided by the carb ratio received from your medical provider. To calculate this amount, use the following as an example:

Meal Carbs (MC) = 120
Correction Factor (CF) = 60

Carb Dose Calculation = MC ÷ CF
= 30 ÷ 16
= **1.875 or 2 units of insulin**
answer rounded to nearest whole number

Ketones - Made when the body is not producing enough insulin.

Use the color chart to keep track of when you check ketone levels with ketone testing strips.

Remember to consult your medical provider with any questions regarding your specific care.

KETONE COLOR CHART

- No Ketones
- Trace Ketones
- Small Ketones
- Moderate Ketones
- Large Ketones
- Large Ketones

EXAMPLE

DATE: February 14, 2026 — SUN MON TUES WED THUR **(FRI)** SAT

	MEALS AND SNACKS	CARB AND FOOD CALCULATIONS	SHOT DETAILS AND LOCATION
BREAKFAST	1½ cup milk 19.5g 1 cup cereal 36g Total Carbohydrates : 55.5 grams	Correction Dose: (BS - 120) / 60 (154-120)/60 = (34/60) = 0.57 Carb Dose Calculation: (Meal Carbs / 16) (55.5 / 16) = 3.47 Correction Dose + Carb Dose Calculation: (0.57 + 3.47) = 4.04 OR 4 UNITS Correction Dose / Dose Calculation / Rounded to nearest whole number	TIME 8 : 45 (AM) / PM LEFT ARM / RIGHT ARM / LEFT LEG / RIGHT LEG / LEFT/RIGHT STOMACH / CGM KETONES: NEGATIVE / TRACE / SMALL / MODERATE / LARGE
SNACK	1 sugar free jello 0g 1 cheese stick 1g 1 Coke Zero 0g Total Carbohydrates : 1.0 grams	Carb Dose Calculation: (Meal Carbs / 16) (1.0 / 16) = 0.06 or — UNITS NO INSULIN DOSE REQUIRED FOR MEALS/SNACKS UNDER 14 G OF CARBS OR EQUAL TO 0.49 OR LESS	TIME 10 : 47 (AM) / PM LEFT ARM / RIGHT ARM / LEFT LEG / RIGHT LEG / LEFT/RIGHT STOMACH / CGM KETONES: NEGATIVE / TRACE / SMALL / MODERATE / LARGE
LUNCH	Ham and cheese sandwich 37g 1 snack chip bag 15g Total Carbohydrates : 52.0 grams	Correction Dose: (BS - 120) / 60 (94-120)/60 = (—/—) = — Carb Dose Calculation: (Meal Carbs / 16) (52.0 / 16) = 3.25 Correction Dose + Carb Dose Calculation: (— + 3.25) = 3.25 OR 3 UNITS Correction Dose / Dose Calculation / Rounded to nearest whole number	TIME 1 : 30 AM / (PM) LEFT ARM / RIGHT ARM / LEFT LEG / RIGHT LEG / LEFT/RIGHT STOMACH / CGM KETONES: NEGATIVE / TRACE / SMALL / MODERATE / LARGE
SNACK	Total Carbohydrates : __._ grams	Carb Dose Calculation: (Meal Carbs / 16) (__._ / ___) = ___.__ or __ UNITS NO INSULIN DOSE REQUIRED FOR MEALS/SNACKS UNDER 14 G OF CARBS OR EQUAL TO 0.49 OR LESS	TIME __ : __ AM / PM LEFT ARM / RIGHT ARM / LEFT LEG / RIGHT LEG / LEFT/RIGHT STOMACH / CGM KETONES: NEGATIVE / TRACE / SMALL / MODERATE / LARGE
DINNER	Small french fries 43g 1 slice of pizza 31.5g Total Carbohydrates : 74.5 grams	Correction Dose: (BS - 120) / 60 (121-120)/60 = (1/60) = 0.02 Carb Dose Calculation: (Meal Carbs / 16) (74.5 / 16) = 4.66 Correction Dose + Carb Dose Calculation: (0.02 + 4.66) = 4.68 OR 5 UNITS Correction Dose / Dose Calculation / Rounded to nearest whole number	TIME 5 : 12 AM / (PM) LEFT ARM / RIGHT ARM / LEFT LEG / RIGHT LEG / LEFT/RIGHT STOMACH / CGM KETONES: NEGATIVE / TRACE / SMALL / MODERATE / LARGE
SNACK	Small cupcake 30g 8oz of sugar free juice 1g Total Carbohydrates : 31.0 grams	Carb Dose Calculation: (Meal Carbs / 16) (31.0 / 16) = 1.94 or 2 UNITS NO INSULIN DOSE REQUIRED FOR MEALS/SNACKS UNDER 14 G OF CARBS OR EQUAL TO 0.49 OR LESS	TIME 7 : 19 AM / (PM) LEFT ARM / RIGHT ARM / LEFT LEG / RIGHT LEG / LEFT/RIGHT STOMACH / CGM KETONES: NEGATIVE / TRACE / SMALL / MODERATE / LARGE

BEDTIME 9 : 00 PM

BLOOD SUGAR 250 — UNITS 19

LEFT ARM / RIGHT ARM / LEFT LEG / RIGHT LEG / LEFT/RIGHT STOMACH / CGM

KETONES: (NEGATIVE) / TRACE / SMALL / MODERATE / LARGE

HYDRATE

2AM BLOOD SUGAR 105

ADDITIONAL BLOOD SUGAR READINGS

BS 183 at 5 : 48 AM/(PM)

BS 200 at 11 : 20 AM/(PM)

NOTES

- New CGM at 5:40pm
- Soccer Practice 6:30pm
- Tylenol at 11:20pm

MEDICINE

- Vitamin D gummy
- Multivitamin gummy

DATE: ______________________ SUN MON TUES WED THUR FRI SAT

	MEALS AND SNACKS	CARB AND FOOD CALCULATIONS	SHOT DETAILS AND LOCATION
BREAKFAST	Total Carbohydrates : ___._ grams	Correction Dose: (BS - ___) / __ (___-___)/__ = (__/__) = ___.__ Carb Dose Calculation: (Meal Carbs / ___) (__._ /___) = ___.__ Correction Dose + Carb Dose Calculation: (___.__ + ___.__) = __.__ OR __ UNITS Correction Dose / Dose Calculation / Rounded to nearest whole number	TIME __:__ AM / PM LEFT ARM CGM / RIGHT ARM CGM / LEFT LEG CGM / RIGHT LEG CGM / LEFT/RIGHT STOMACH CGM KETONES NEGATIVE / TRACE / SMALL / MODERATE / LARGE
SNACK	Total Carbohydrates : ___._ grams	Carb Dose Calculation: (Meal Carbs / ___) (__._ /___) = ___.__ or __ UNITS NO INSULIN DOSE REQUIRED FOR MEALS/SNACKS UNDER __G OF CARBS OR EQUAL TO __.__ OR LESS	TIME __:__ AM / PM LEFT ARM CGM / RIGHT ARM CGM / LEFT LEG CGM / RIGHT LEG CGM / LEFT/RIGHT STOMACH CGM KETONES NEGATIVE / TRACE / SMALL / MODERATE / LARGE
LUNCH	Total Carbohydrates : ___._ grams	Correction Dose: (BS - ___) / __ (___-___)/__ = (__/__) = ___.__ Carb Dose Calculation: (Meal Carbs / ___) (__._ /___) = ___.__ Correction Dose + Carb Dose Calculation: (___.__ + ___.__) = __.__ OR __ UNITS Correction Dose / Dose Calculation / Rounded to nearest whole number	TIME __:__ AM / PM LEFT ARM CGM / RIGHT ARM CGM / LEFT LEG CGM / RIGHT LEG CGM / LEFT/RIGHT STOMACH CGM KETONES NEGATIVE / TRACE / SMALL / MODERATE / LARGE
SNACK	Total Carbohydrates : ___._ grams	Carb Dose Calculation: (Meal Carbs / ___) (__._ /___) = ___.__ or __ UNITS NO INSULIN DOSE REQUIRED FOR MEALS/SNACKS UNDER __G OF CARBS OR EQUAL TO __.__ OR LESS	TIME __:__ AM / PM LEFT ARM CGM / RIGHT ARM CGM / LEFT LEG CGM / RIGHT LEG CGM / LEFT/RIGHT STOMACH CGM KETONES NEGATIVE / TRACE / SMALL / MODERATE / LARGE
DINNER	Total Carbohydrates : ___._ grams	Correction Dose: (BS - ___) / __ (___-___)/__ = (__/__) = ___.__ Carb Dose Calculation: (Meal Carbs / ___) (__._ /___) = ___.__ Correction Dose + Carb Dose Calculation: (___.__ + ___.__) = __.__ OR __ UNITS Correction Dose / Dose Calculation / Rounded to nearest whole number	TIME __:__ AM / PM LEFT ARM CGM / RIGHT ARM CGM / LEFT LEG CGM / RIGHT LEG CGM / LEFT/RIGHT STOMACH CGM KETONES NEGATIVE / TRACE / SMALL / MODERATE / LARGE
SNACK	Total Carbohydrates : ___._ grams	Carb Dose Calculation: (Meal Carbs / ___) (__._ /___) = ___.__ or __ UNITS NO INSULIN DOSE REQUIRED FOR MEALS/SNACKS UNDER __G OF CARBS OR EQUAL TO __.__ OR LESS	TIME __:__ AM / PM LEFT ARM CGM / RIGHT ARM CGM / LEFT LEG CGM / RIGHT LEG CGM / LEFT/RIGHT STOMACH CGM KETONES NEGATIVE / TRACE / SMALL / MODERATE / LARGE
BEDTIME __:__ PM	BLOOD SUGAR ____ UNITS ___ LEFT ARM CGM / RIGHT ARM CGM / LEFT LEG CGM / RIGHT LEG CGM / LEFT/RIGHT STOMACH CGM KETONES NEGATIVE / TRACE / SMALL / MODERATE / LARGE	HYDRATE 2AM BLOOD SUGAR ____ ADDITIONAL BLOOD SUGAR READINGS BS ___ at __ : __ AM/PM BS ___ at __ : __ AM/PM	NOTES MEDICINE

DATE: ______________________________ SUN MON TUES WED THUR FRI SAT

	MEALS AND SNACKS	CARB AND FOOD CALCULATIONS	SHOT DETAILS AND LOCATION
BREAKFAST	Total Carbohydrates : ___._ grams	Correction Dose: (BS - ___) / __ (___-___)/__ = (__/__) = ___.__ Carb Dose Calculation: (Meal Carbs / ___) (__._ /___) = ___.__ Correction Dose + Carb Dose Calculation: (__.__ + __.__) = __.__ OR __ UNITS Correction Dose · Dose Calculation · Rounded to nearest whole number	TIME __ : __ AM / PM LEFT ARM CGM · RIGHT ARM CGM · LEFT LEG CGM · RIGHT LEG CGM · LEFT/RIGHT STOMACH CGM KETONES NEGATIVE · TRACE · SMALL · MODERATE · LARGE
SNACK	Total Carbohydrates : ___._ grams	Carb Dose Calculation: (Meal Carbs / ___) (__._ /___) = ___.__ or __ UNITS NO INSULIN DOSE REQUIRED FOR MEALS/SNACKS UNDER __G OF CARBS OR EQUAL TO __.__ OR LESS	TIME __ : __ AM / PM LEFT ARM CGM · RIGHT ARM CGM · LEFT LEG CGM · RIGHT LEG CGM · LEFT/RIGHT STOMACH CGM KETONES NEGATIVE · TRACE · SMALL · MODERATE · LARGE
LUNCH	Total Carbohydrates : ___._ grams	Correction Dose: (BS - ___) / __ (___-___)/__ = (__/__) = ___.__ Carb Dose Calculation: (Meal Carbs / ___) (__._ /___) = ___.__ Correction Dose + Carb Dose Calculation: (__.__ + __.__) = __.__ OR __ UNITS Correction Dose · Dose Calculation · Rounded to nearest whole number	TIME __ : __ AM / PM LEFT ARM CGM · RIGHT ARM CGM · LEFT LEG CGM · RIGHT LEG CGM · LEFT/RIGHT STOMACH CGM KETONES NEGATIVE · TRACE · SMALL · MODERATE · LARGE
SNACK	Total Carbohydrates : ___._ grams	Carb Dose Calculation: (Meal Carbs / ___) (__._ /___) = ___.__ or __ UNITS NO INSULIN DOSE REQUIRED FOR MEALS/SNACKS UNDER __G OF CARBS OR EQUAL TO __.__ OR LESS	TIME __ : __ AM / PM LEFT ARM CGM · RIGHT ARM CGM · LEFT LEG CGM · RIGHT LEG CGM · LEFT/RIGHT STOMACH CGM KETONES NEGATIVE · TRACE · SMALL · MODERATE · LARGE
DINNER	Total Carbohydrates : ___._ grams	Correction Dose: (BS - ___) / __ (___-___)/__ = (__/__) = ___.__ Carb Dose Calculation: (Meal Carbs / ___) (__._ /___) = ___.__ Correction Dose + Carb Dose Calculation: (__.__ + __.__) = __.__ OR __ UNITS Correction Dose · Dose Calculation · Rounded to nearest whole number	TIME __ : __ AM / PM LEFT ARM CGM · RIGHT ARM CGM · LEFT LEG CGM · RIGHT LEG CGM · LEFT/RIGHT STOMACH CGM KETONES NEGATIVE · TRACE · SMALL · MODERATE · LARGE
SNACK	Total Carbohydrates : ___._ grams	Carb Dose Calculation: (Meal Carbs / ___) (__._ /___) = ___.__ or __ UNITS NO INSULIN DOSE REQUIRED FOR MEALS/SNACKS UNDER __G OF CARBS OR EQUAL TO __.__ OR LESS	TIME __ : __ AM / PM LEFT ARM CGM · RIGHT ARM CGM · LEFT LEG CGM · RIGHT LEG CGM · LEFT/RIGHT STOMACH CGM KETONES NEGATIVE · TRACE · SMALL · MODERATE · LARGE
BEDTIME __ : __ PM	BLOOD SUGAR ____ UNITS ___ LEFT ARM CGM · RIGHT ARM CGM · LEFT LEG CGM · RIGHT LEG CGM · LEFT/RIGHT STOMACH CGM KETONES NEGATIVE · TRACE · SMALL · MODERATE · LARGE	HYDRATE 2AM BLOOD SUGAR ____ ADDITIONAL BLOOD SUGAR READINGS BS ___ at __ : __ AM/PM BS ___ at __ : __ AM/PM	NOTES MEDICINE

DATE: ______________________________ SUN MON TUES WED THUR FRI SAT

	MEALS AND SNACKS	CARB AND FOOD CALCULATIONS	SHOT DETAILS AND LOCATION
BREAKFAST	Total Carbohydrates : ___._ grams	Correction Dose: (BS - ___) / __ (___-___)/__ = (__/__) = ___.__ Carb Dose Calculation: (Meal Carbs / ___) (__._ /___) = ___.__ Correction Dose + Carb Dose Calculation: (__.__ + __.__) = __.__ OR __ UNITS Correction Dose / Dose Calculation / Rounded to nearest whole number	TIME __ : __ AM / PM LEFT ARM CGM / RIGHT ARM CGM / LEFT LEG CGM / RIGHT LEG CGM / LEFT/RIGHT STOMACH CGM KETONES NEGATIVE / TRACE / SMALL / MODERATE / LARGE
SNACK	Total Carbohydrates : ___._ grams	Carb Dose Calculation: (Meal Carbs / ___) (__._ /___) = ___.__ or __ UNITS NO INSULIN DOSE REQUIRED FOR MEALS/SNACKS UNDER __G OF CARBS OR EQUAL TO __.__ OR LESS	TIME __ : __ AM / PM LEFT ARM CGM / RIGHT ARM CGM / LEFT LEG CGM / RIGHT LEG CGM / LEFT/RIGHT STOMACH CGM KETONES NEGATIVE / TRACE / SMALL / MODERATE / LARGE
LUNCH	Total Carbohydrates : ___._ grams	Correction Dose: (BS - ___) / __ (___-___)/__ = (__/__) = ___.__ Carb Dose Calculation: (Meal Carbs / ___) (__._ /___) = ___.__ Correction Dose + Carb Dose Calculation: (__.__ + __.__) = __.__ OR __ UNITS Correction Dose / Dose Calculation / Rounded to nearest whole number	TIME __ : __ AM / PM LEFT ARM CGM / RIGHT ARM CGM / LEFT LEG CGM / RIGHT LEG CGM / LEFT/RIGHT STOMACH CGM KETONES NEGATIVE / TRACE / SMALL / MODERATE / LARGE
SNACK	Total Carbohydrates : ___._ grams	Carb Dose Calculation: (Meal Carbs / ___) (__._ /___) = ___.__ or __ UNITS NO INSULIN DOSE REQUIRED FOR MEALS/SNACKS UNDER __G OF CARBS OR EQUAL TO __.__ OR LESS	TIME __ : __ AM / PM LEFT ARM CGM / RIGHT ARM CGM / LEFT LEG CGM / RIGHT LEG CGM / LEFT/RIGHT STOMACH CGM KETONES NEGATIVE / TRACE / SMALL / MODERATE / LARGE
DINNER	Total Carbohydrates : ___._ grams	Correction Dose: (BS - ___) / __ (___-___)/__ = (__/__) = ___.__ Carb Dose Calculation: (Meal Carbs / ___) (__._ /___) = ___.__ Correction Dose + Carb Dose Calculation: (__.__ + __.__) = __.__ OR __ UNITS Correction Dose / Dose Calculation / Rounded to nearest whole number	TIME __ : __ AM / PM LEFT ARM CGM / RIGHT ARM CGM / LEFT LEG CGM / RIGHT LEG CGM / LEFT/RIGHT STOMACH CGM KETONES NEGATIVE / TRACE / SMALL / MODERATE / LARGE
SNACK	Total Carbohydrates : ___._ grams	Carb Dose Calculation: (Meal Carbs / ___) (__._ /___) = ___.__ or __ UNITS NO INSULIN DOSE REQUIRED FOR MEALS/SNACKS UNDER __G OF CARBS OR EQUAL TO __.__ OR LESS	TIME __ : __ AM / PM LEFT ARM CGM / RIGHT ARM CGM / LEFT LEG CGM / RIGHT LEG CGM / LEFT/RIGHT STOMACH CGM KETONES NEGATIVE / TRACE / SMALL / MODERATE / LARGE
BEDTIME __ : __ PM	BLOOD SUGAR _____ UNITS ___ LEFT ARM CGM / RIGHT ARM CGM / LEFT LEG CGM / RIGHT LEG CGM / LEFT/RIGHT STOMACH CGM KETONES NEGATIVE / TRACE / SMALL / MODERATE / LARGE	HYDRATE 2AM BLOOD SUGAR _____ ADDITIONAL BLOOD SUGAR READINGS BS ___ at __ : __ AM/PM BS ___ at __ : __ AM/PM	NOTES MEDICINE

DATE: ______________________________ SUN MON TUES WED THUR FRI SAT

	MEALS AND SNACKS	CARB AND FOOD CALCULATIONS	SHOT DETAILS AND LOCATION
BREAKFAST	Total Carbohydrates : ___._ grams	Correction Dose: (BS - ___) / __ (___-___)/__ = (__/__) = ___.__ Carb Dose Calculation: (Meal Carbs / ___) (__._ /___) = ___.__ Correction Dose + Carb Dose Calculation: (___.__ + ___.__) = __.__ OR __ UNITS Correction Dose / Dose Calculation / Rounded to nearest whole number	TIME __ : __ AM / PM LEFT ARM CGM / RIGHT ARM CGM / LEFT LEG CGM / RIGHT LEG CGM / LEFT/RIGHT STOMACH CGM KETONES NEGATIVE TRACE SMALL MODERATE LARGE
SNACK	Total Carbohydrates : ___._ grams	Carb Dose Calculation: (Meal Carbs / ___) (__._ /___) = ___.__ or __ UNITS NO INSULIN DOSE REQUIRED FOR MEALS/SNACKS UNDER __G OF CARBS OR EQUAL TO __.__ OR LESS	TIME __ : __ AM / PM LEFT ARM CGM / RIGHT ARM CGM / LEFT LEG CGM / RIGHT LEG CGM / LEFT/RIGHT STOMACH CGM KETONES NEGATIVE TRACE SMALL MODERATE LARGE
LUNCH	Total Carbohydrates : ___._ grams	Correction Dose: (BS - ___) / __ (___-___)/__ = (__/__) = ___.__ Carb Dose Calculation: (Meal Carbs / ___) (__._ /___) = ___.__ Correction Dose + Carb Dose Calculation: (___.__ + ___.__) = __.__ OR __ UNITS Correction Dose / Dose Calculation / Rounded to nearest whole number	TIME __ : __ AM / PM LEFT ARM CGM / RIGHT ARM CGM / LEFT LEG CGM / RIGHT LEG CGM / LEFT/RIGHT STOMACH CGM KETONES NEGATIVE TRACE SMALL MODERATE LARGE
SNACK	Total Carbohydrates : ___._ grams	Carb Dose Calculation: (Meal Carbs / ___) (__._ /___) = ___.__ or __ UNITS NO INSULIN DOSE REQUIRED FOR MEALS/SNACKS UNDER __G OF CARBS OR EQUAL TO __.__ OR LESS	TIME __ : __ AM / PM LEFT ARM CGM / RIGHT ARM CGM / LEFT LEG CGM / RIGHT LEG CGM / LEFT/RIGHT STOMACH CGM KETONES NEGATIVE TRACE SMALL MODERATE LARGE
DINNER	Total Carbohydrates : ___._ grams	Correction Dose: (BS - ___) / __ (___-___)/__ = (__/__) = ___.__ Carb Dose Calculation: (Meal Carbs / ___) (__._ /___) = ___.__ Correction Dose + Carb Dose Calculation: (___.__ + ___.__) = __.__ OR __ UNITS Correction Dose / Dose Calculation / Rounded to nearest whole number	TIME __ : __ AM / PM LEFT ARM CGM / RIGHT ARM CGM / LEFT LEG CGM / RIGHT LEG CGM / LEFT/RIGHT STOMACH CGM KETONES NEGATIVE TRACE SMALL MODERATE LARGE
SNACK	Total Carbohydrates : ___._ grams	Carb Dose Calculation: (Meal Carbs / ___) (__._ /___) = ___.__ or __ UNITS NO INSULIN DOSE REQUIRED FOR MEALS/SNACKS UNDER __G OF CARBS OR EQUAL TO __.__ OR LESS	TIME __ : __ AM / PM LEFT ARM CGM / RIGHT ARM CGM / LEFT LEG CGM / RIGHT LEG CGM / LEFT/RIGHT STOMACH CGM KETONES NEGATIVE TRACE SMALL MODERATE LARGE
BEDTIME __ : __ PM	BLOOD SUGAR ____ UNITS ___ LEFT ARM CGM / RIGHT ARM CGM / LEFT LEG CGM / RIGHT LEG CGM / LEFT/RIGHT STOMACH CGM KETONES NEGATIVE TRACE SMALL MODERATE LARGE	HYDRATE 2AM BLOOD SUGAR ____ ADDITIONAL BLOOD SUGAR READINGS BS ___ at __ : __ AM/PM BS ___ at __ : __ AM/PM	NOTES MEDICINE

DATE: ____________________ SUN MON TUES WED THUR FRI SAT

	MEALS AND SNACKS	CARB AND FOOD CALCULATIONS	SHOT DETAILS AND LOCATION
BREAKFAST	Total Carbohydrates : ___._ grams	Correction Dose: (BS - ___) / __ (___-___)/__ = (__/__) = ___.__ Carb Dose Calculation: (Meal Carbs / ___) (__._ /___) = ___.__ Correction Dose + Carb Dose Calculation: (___.__ + ___.__) = __.__ OR __ UNITS Correction Dose / Dose Calculation / Rounded to nearest whole number	TIME __ : __ AM / PM LEFT ARM CGM / RIGHT ARM CGM / LEFT LEG CGM / RIGHT LEG CGM / LEFT/RIGHT STOMACH CGM KETONES NEGATIVE / TRACE / SMALL / MODERATE / LARGE
SNACK	Total Carbohydrates : ___._ grams	Carb Dose Calculation: (Meal Carbs / ___) (__._ /___) = ___.__ or __ UNITS NO INSULIN DOSE REQUIRED FOR MEALS/SNACKS UNDER __G OF CARBS OR EQUAL TO __.__ OR LESS	TIME __ : __ AM / PM LEFT ARM CGM / RIGHT ARM CGM / LEFT LEG CGM / RIGHT LEG CGM / LEFT/RIGHT STOMACH CGM KETONES NEGATIVE / TRACE / SMALL / MODERATE / LARGE
LUNCH	Total Carbohydrates : ___._ grams	Correction Dose: (BS - ___) / __ (___-___)/__ = (__/__) = ___.__ Carb Dose Calculation: (Meal Carbs / ___) (__._ /___) = ___.__ Correction Dose + Carb Dose Calculation: (___.__ + ___.__) = __.__ OR __ UNITS Correction Dose / Dose Calculation / Rounded to nearest whole number	TIME __ : __ AM / PM LEFT ARM CGM / RIGHT ARM CGM / LEFT LEG CGM / RIGHT LEG CGM / LEFT/RIGHT STOMACH CGM KETONES NEGATIVE / TRACE / SMALL / MODERATE / LARGE
SNACK	Total Carbohydrates : ___._ grams	Carb Dose Calculation: (Meal Carbs / ___) (__._ /___) = ___.__ or __ UNITS NO INSULIN DOSE REQUIRED FOR MEALS/SNACKS UNDER __G OF CARBS OR EQUAL TO __.__ OR LESS	TIME __ : __ AM / PM LEFT ARM CGM / RIGHT ARM CGM / LEFT LEG CGM / RIGHT LEG CGM / LEFT/RIGHT STOMACH CGM KETONES NEGATIVE / TRACE / SMALL / MODERATE / LARGE
DINNER	Total Carbohydrates : ___._ grams	Correction Dose: (BS - ___) / __ (___-___)/__ = (__/__) = ___.__ Carb Dose Calculation: (Meal Carbs / ___) (__._ /___) = ___.__ Correction Dose + Carb Dose Calculation: (___.__ + ___.__) = __.__ OR __ UNITS Correction Dose / Dose Calculation / Rounded to nearest whole number	TIME __ : __ AM / PM LEFT ARM CGM / RIGHT ARM CGM / LEFT LEG CGM / RIGHT LEG CGM / LEFT/RIGHT STOMACH CGM KETONES NEGATIVE / TRACE / SMALL / MODERATE / LARGE
SNACK	Total Carbohydrates : ___._ grams	Carb Dose Calculation: (Meal Carbs / ___) (__._ /___) = ___.__ or __ UNITS NO INSULIN DOSE REQUIRED FOR MEALS/SNACKS UNDER __G OF CARBS OR EQUAL TO __.__ OR LESS	TIME __ : __ AM / PM LEFT ARM CGM / RIGHT ARM CGM / LEFT LEG CGM / RIGHT LEG CGM / LEFT/RIGHT STOMACH CGM KETONES NEGATIVE / TRACE / SMALL / MODERATE / LARGE
BEDTIME __ : __ PM	BLOOD SUGAR _____ UNITS ___ LEFT ARM CGM / RIGHT ARM CGM / LEFT LEG CGM / RIGHT LEG CGM / LEFT/RIGHT STOMACH CGM KETONES NEGATIVE / TRACE / SMALL / MODERATE / LARGE	HYDRATE 2AM BLOOD SUGAR _____ ADDITIONAL BLOOD SUGAR READINGS BS ___ at __ : __ AM/PM BS ___ at __ : __ AM/PM	NOTES MEDICINE

DATE: ____________________ SUN MON TUES WED THUR FRI SAT

	MEALS AND SNACKS	CARB AND FOOD CALCULATIONS	SHOT DETAILS AND LOCATION
BREAKFAST	Total Carbohydrates : ___._ grams	Correction Dose: (BS - ___) / __ (___-___)/__ = (__/__) = ___.__ Carb Dose Calculation: (Meal Carbs / ___) (__._ /___) = ___.__ Correction Dose + Carb Dose Calculation: (___.__ + ___.__) = __.__ OR __ UNITS Correction Dose / Dose Calculation / Rounded to nearest whole number	TIME __ : __ AM / PM LEFT ARM CGM / RIGHT ARM CGM / LEFT LEG CGM / RIGHT LEG CGM / LEFT/RIGHT STOMACH CGM KETONES NEGATIVE TRACE SMALL MODERATE LARGE
SNACK	Total Carbohydrates : ___._ grams	Carb Dose Calculation: (Meal Carbs / ___) (__._ /___) = ___.__ or __ UNITS NO INSULIN DOSE REQUIRED FOR MEALS/SNACKS UNDER __G OF CARBS OR EQUAL TO __.__ OR LESS	TIME __ : __ AM / PM LEFT ARM CGM / RIGHT ARM CGM / LEFT LEG CGM / RIGHT LEG CGM / LEFT/RIGHT STOMACH CGM KETONES NEGATIVE TRACE SMALL MODERATE LARGE
LUNCH	Total Carbohydrates : ___._ grams	Correction Dose: (BS - ___) / __ (___-___)/__ = (__/__) = ___.__ Carb Dose Calculation: (Meal Carbs / ___) (__._ /___) = ___.__ Correction Dose + Carb Dose Calculation: (___.__ + ___.__) = __.__ OR __ UNITS Correction Dose / Dose Calculation / Rounded to nearest whole number	TIME __ : __ AM / PM LEFT ARM CGM / RIGHT ARM CGM / LEFT LEG CGM / RIGHT LEG CGM / LEFT/RIGHT STOMACH CGM KETONES NEGATIVE TRACE SMALL MODERATE LARGE
SNACK	Total Carbohydrates : ___._ grams	Carb Dose Calculation: (Meal Carbs / ___) (__._ /___) = ___.__ or __ UNITS NO INSULIN DOSE REQUIRED FOR MEALS/SNACKS UNDER __G OF CARBS OR EQUAL TO __.__ OR LESS	TIME __ : __ AM / PM LEFT ARM CGM / RIGHT ARM CGM / LEFT LEG CGM / RIGHT LEG CGM / LEFT/RIGHT STOMACH CGM KETONES NEGATIVE TRACE SMALL MODERATE LARGE
DINNER	Total Carbohydrates : ___._ grams	Correction Dose: (BS - ___) / __ (___-___)/__ = (__/__) = ___.__ Carb Dose Calculation: (Meal Carbs / ___) (__._ /___) = ___.__ Correction Dose + Carb Dose Calculation: (___.__ + ___.__) = __.__ OR __ UNITS Correction Dose / Dose Calculation / Rounded to nearest whole number	TIME __ : __ AM / PM LEFT ARM CGM / RIGHT ARM CGM / LEFT LEG CGM / RIGHT LEG CGM / LEFT/RIGHT STOMACH CGM KETONES NEGATIVE TRACE SMALL MODERATE LARGE
SNACK	Total Carbohydrates : ___._ grams	Carb Dose Calculation: (Meal Carbs / ___) (__._ /___) = ___.__ or __ UNITS NO INSULIN DOSE REQUIRED FOR MEALS/SNACKS UNDER __G OF CARBS OR EQUAL TO __.__ OR LESS	TIME __ : __ AM / PM LEFT ARM CGM / RIGHT ARM CGM / LEFT LEG CGM / RIGHT LEG CGM / LEFT/RIGHT STOMACH CGM KETONES NEGATIVE TRACE SMALL MODERATE LARGE
BEDTIME __ : __ PM	BLOOD SUGAR _____ UNITS ___ LEFT ARM CGM / RIGHT ARM CGM / LEFT LEG CGM / RIGHT LEG CGM / LEFT/RIGHT STOMACH CGM KETONES NEGATIVE TRACE SMALL MODERATE LARGE	HYDRATE 2AM BLOOD SUGAR _____ ADDITIONAL BLOOD SUGAR READINGS BS ___ at __ : __ AM/PM BS ___ at __ : __ AM/PM	NOTES MEDICINE

DATE: ______________________ SUN MON TUES WED THUR FRI SAT

	MEALS AND SNACKS	CARB AND FOOD CALCULATIONS	SHOT DETAILS AND LOCATION
BREAKFAST	Total Carbohydrates : ___._ grams	Correction Dose: (BS - ___) / __ (___-___)/__ = (__/__) = ___.__ Carb Dose Calculation: (Meal Carbs / ___) (__._ /___) = ___.__ Correction Dose + Carb Dose Calculation: (__.__ + __.__) = __.__ OR __ UNITS Correction Dose / Dose Calculation / Rounded to nearest whole number	TIME __ : __ AM / PM LEFT ARM CGM / RIGHT ARM CGM / LEFT LEG CGM / RIGHT LEG CGM / LEFT/RIGHT STOMACH CGM KETONES NEGATIVE TRACE SMALL MODERATE LARGE
SNACK	Total Carbohydrates : ___._ grams	Carb Dose Calculation: (Meal Carbs / ___) (__._ /___) = ___.__ or __ UNITS NO INSULIN DOSE REQUIRED FOR MEALS/SNACKS UNDER __G OF CARBS OR EQUAL TO __.__ OR LESS	TIME __ : __ AM / PM LEFT ARM CGM / RIGHT ARM CGM / LEFT LEG CGM / RIGHT LEG CGM / LEFT/RIGHT STOMACH CGM KETONES NEGATIVE TRACE SMALL MODERATE LARGE
LUNCH	Total Carbohydrates : ___._ grams	Correction Dose: (BS - ___) / __ (___-___)/__ = (__/__) = ___.__ Carb Dose Calculation: (Meal Carbs / ___) (__._ /___) = ___.__ Correction Dose + Carb Dose Calculation: (__.__ + __.__) = __.__ OR __ UNITS Correction Dose / Dose Calculation / Rounded to nearest whole number	TIME __ : __ AM / PM LEFT ARM CGM / RIGHT ARM CGM / LEFT LEG CGM / RIGHT LEG CGM / LEFT/RIGHT STOMACH CGM KETONES NEGATIVE TRACE SMALL MODERATE LARGE
SNACK	Total Carbohydrates : ___._ grams	Carb Dose Calculation: (Meal Carbs / ___) (__._ /___) = ___.__ or __ UNITS NO INSULIN DOSE REQUIRED FOR MEALS/SNACKS UNDER __G OF CARBS OR EQUAL TO __.__ OR LESS	TIME __ : __ AM / PM LEFT ARM CGM / RIGHT ARM CGM / LEFT LEG CGM / RIGHT LEG CGM / LEFT/RIGHT STOMACH CGM KETONES NEGATIVE TRACE SMALL MODERATE LARGE
DINNER	Total Carbohydrates : ___._ grams	Correction Dose: (BS - ___) / __ (___-___)/__ = (__/__) = ___.__ Carb Dose Calculation: (Meal Carbs / ___) (__._ /___) = ___.__ Correction Dose + Carb Dose Calculation: (__.__ + __.__) = __.__ OR __ UNITS Correction Dose / Dose Calculation / Rounded to nearest whole number	TIME __ : __ AM / PM LEFT ARM CGM / RIGHT ARM CGM / LEFT LEG CGM / RIGHT LEG CGM / LEFT/RIGHT STOMACH CGM KETONES NEGATIVE TRACE SMALL MODERATE LARGE
SNACK	Total Carbohydrates : ___._ grams	Carb Dose Calculation: (Meal Carbs / ___) (__._ /___) = ___.__ or __ UNITS NO INSULIN DOSE REQUIRED FOR MEALS/SNACKS UNDER __G OF CARBS OR EQUAL TO __.__ OR LESS	TIME __ : __ AM / PM LEFT ARM CGM / RIGHT ARM CGM / LEFT LEG CGM / RIGHT LEG CGM / LEFT/RIGHT STOMACH CGM KETONES NEGATIVE TRACE SMALL MODERATE LARGE
BEDTIME __ : __ PM	BLOOD SUGAR ____ UNITS ___ LEFT ARM CGM / RIGHT ARM CGM / LEFT LEG CGM / RIGHT LEG CGM / LEFT/RIGHT STOMACH CGM KETONES NEGATIVE TRACE SMALL MODERATE LARGE	HYDRATE 2AM BLOOD SUGAR ____ ADDITIONAL BLOOD SUGAR READINGS BS ___ at __ : __ AM/PM BS ___ at __ : __ AM/PM	NOTES MEDICINE

DATE: ______________________________ SUN MON TUES WED THUR FRI SAT

	MEALS AND SNACKS	CARB AND FOOD CALCULATIONS	SHOT DETAILS AND LOCATION
BREAKFAST	Total Carbohydrates : ___._ grams	Correction Dose: (BS - ___) / __ (___-___)/__ = (__/__) = ___.__ Carb Dose Calculation: (Meal Carbs / ___) (__._ /___) = ___.__ Correction Dose + Carb Dose Calculation: (__.__ + __.__) = __.__ OR __ UNITS Correction Dose / Dose Calculation / Rounded to nearest whole number	TIME __ : __ AM / PM LEFT ARM CGM / RIGHT ARM CGM / LEFT LEG CGM / RIGHT LEG CGM / LEFT/RIGHT STOMACH CGM KETONES NEGATIVE / TRACE / SMALL / MODERATE / LARGE
SNACK	Total Carbohydrates : ___._ grams	Carb Dose Calculation: (Meal Carbs / ___) (__._ /___) = ___.__ or __ UNITS NO INSULIN DOSE REQUIRED FOR MEALS/SNACKS UNDER __G OF CARBS OR EQUAL TO __.__ OR LESS	TIME __ : __ AM / PM LEFT ARM CGM / RIGHT ARM CGM / LEFT LEG CGM / RIGHT LEG CGM / LEFT/RIGHT STOMACH CGM KETONES NEGATIVE / TRACE / SMALL / MODERATE / LARGE
LUNCH	Total Carbohydrates : ___._ grams	Correction Dose: (BS - ___) / __ (___-___)/__ = (__/__) = ___.__ Carb Dose Calculation: (Meal Carbs / ___) (__._ /___) = ___.__ Correction Dose + Carb Dose Calculation: (__.__ + __.__) = __.__ OR __ UNITS Correction Dose / Dose Calculation / Rounded to nearest whole number	TIME __ : __ AM / PM LEFT ARM CGM / RIGHT ARM CGM / LEFT LEG CGM / RIGHT LEG CGM / LEFT/RIGHT STOMACH CGM KETONES NEGATIVE / TRACE / SMALL / MODERATE / LARGE
SNACK	Total Carbohydrates : ___._ grams	Carb Dose Calculation: (Meal Carbs / ___) (__._ /___) = ___.__ or __ UNITS NO INSULIN DOSE REQUIRED FOR MEALS/SNACKS UNDER __G OF CARBS OR EQUAL TO __.__ OR LESS	TIME __ : __ AM / PM LEFT ARM CGM / RIGHT ARM CGM / LEFT LEG CGM / RIGHT LEG CGM / LEFT/RIGHT STOMACH CGM KETONES NEGATIVE / TRACE / SMALL / MODERATE / LARGE
DINNER	Total Carbohydrates : ___._ grams	Correction Dose: (BS - ___) / __ (___-___)/__ = (__/__) = ___.__ Carb Dose Calculation: (Meal Carbs / ___) (__._ /___) = ___.__ Correction Dose + Carb Dose Calculation: (__.__ + __.__) = __.__ OR __ UNITS Correction Dose / Dose Calculation / Rounded to nearest whole number	TIME __ : __ AM / PM LEFT ARM CGM / RIGHT ARM CGM / LEFT LEG CGM / RIGHT LEG CGM / LEFT/RIGHT STOMACH CGM KETONES NEGATIVE / TRACE / SMALL / MODERATE / LARGE
SNACK	Total Carbohydrates : ___._ grams	Carb Dose Calculation: (Meal Carbs / ___) (__._ /___) = ___.__ or __ UNITS NO INSULIN DOSE REQUIRED FOR MEALS/SNACKS UNDER __G OF CARBS OR EQUAL TO __.__ OR LESS	TIME __ : __ AM / PM LEFT ARM CGM / RIGHT ARM CGM / LEFT LEG CGM / RIGHT LEG CGM / LEFT/RIGHT STOMACH CGM KETONES NEGATIVE / TRACE / SMALL / MODERATE / LARGE
BEDTIME __ : __ PM	BLOOD SUGAR ____ UNITS ___ LEFT ARM CGM / RIGHT ARM CGM / LEFT LEG CGM / RIGHT LEG CGM / LEFT/RIGHT STOMACH CGM KETONES NEGATIVE / TRACE / SMALL / MODERATE / LARGE	HYDRATE 2AM BLOOD SUGAR ____ ADDITIONAL BLOOD SUGAR READINGS BS ___ at __ : __ AM/PM BS ___ at __ : __ AM/PM	NOTES MEDICINE

DATE: ______________________________ SUN MON TUES WED THUR FRI SAT

	MEALS AND SNACKS	CARB AND FOOD CALCULATIONS	SHOT DETAILS AND LOCATION
BREAKFAST	Total Carbohydrates : ___._ grams	Correction Dose: (BS - ___) / __ (___-___)/__ = (__/__) = ___.__ Carb Dose Calculation: (Meal Carbs / ___) (__._ /___) = ___.__ Correction Dose + Carb Dose Calculation: (__.__ + __.__) = __.__ OR __ UNITS Correction Dose · Dose Calculation · Rounded to nearest whole number	TIME __ : __ AM / PM LEFT ARM CGM · RIGHT ARM CGM · LEFT LEG CGM · RIGHT LEG CGM · LEFT/RIGHT STOMACH CGM KETONES NEGATIVE · TRACE · SMALL · MODERATE · LARGE
SNACK	Total Carbohydrates : ___._ grams	Carb Dose Calculation: (Meal Carbs / ___) (__._ /___) = ___.__ or __ UNITS NO INSULIN DOSE REQUIRED FOR MEALS/SNACKS UNDER __G OF CARBS OR EQUAL TO __.__ OR LESS	TIME __ : __ AM / PM LEFT ARM CGM · RIGHT ARM CGM · LEFT LEG CGM · RIGHT LEG CGM · LEFT/RIGHT STOMACH CGM KETONES NEGATIVE · TRACE · SMALL · MODERATE · LARGE
LUNCH	Total Carbohydrates : ___._ grams	Correction Dose: (BS - ___) / __ (___-___)/__ = (__/__) = ___.__ Carb Dose Calculation: (Meal Carbs / ___) (__._ /___) = ___.__ Correction Dose + Carb Dose Calculation: (__.__ + __.__) = __.__ OR __ UNITS Correction Dose · Dose Calculation · Rounded to nearest whole number	TIME __ : __ AM / PM LEFT ARM CGM · RIGHT ARM CGM · LEFT LEG CGM · RIGHT LEG CGM · LEFT/RIGHT STOMACH CGM KETONES NEGATIVE · TRACE · SMALL · MODERATE · LARGE
SNACK	Total Carbohydrates : ___._ grams	Carb Dose Calculation: (Meal Carbs / ___) (__._ /___) = ___.__ or __ UNITS NO INSULIN DOSE REQUIRED FOR MEALS/SNACKS UNDER __G OF CARBS OR EQUAL TO __.__ OR LESS	TIME __ : __ AM / PM LEFT ARM CGM · RIGHT ARM CGM · LEFT LEG CGM · RIGHT LEG CGM · LEFT/RIGHT STOMACH CGM KETONES NEGATIVE · TRACE · SMALL · MODERATE · LARGE
DINNER	Total Carbohydrates : ___._ grams	Correction Dose: (BS - ___) / __ (___-___)/__ = (__/__) = ___.__ Carb Dose Calculation: (Meal Carbs / ___) (__._ /___) = ___.__ Correction Dose + Carb Dose Calculation: (__.__ + __.__) = __.__ OR __ UNITS Correction Dose · Dose Calculation · Rounded to nearest whole number	TIME __ : __ AM / PM LEFT ARM CGM · RIGHT ARM CGM · LEFT LEG CGM · RIGHT LEG CGM · LEFT/RIGHT STOMACH CGM KETONES NEGATIVE · TRACE · SMALL · MODERATE · LARGE
SNACK	Total Carbohydrates : ___._ grams	Carb Dose Calculation: (Meal Carbs / ___) (__._ /___) = ___.__ or __ UNITS NO INSULIN DOSE REQUIRED FOR MEALS/SNACKS UNDER __G OF CARBS OR EQUAL TO __.__ OR LESS	TIME __ : __ AM / PM LEFT ARM CGM · RIGHT ARM CGM · LEFT LEG CGM · RIGHT LEG CGM · LEFT/RIGHT STOMACH CGM KETONES NEGATIVE · TRACE · SMALL · MODERATE · LARGE
BEDTIME __ : __ PM	BLOOD SUGAR _____ UNITS ___ LEFT ARM CGM · RIGHT ARM CGM · LEFT LEG CGM · RIGHT LEG CGM · LEFT/RIGHT STOMACH CGM KETONES NEGATIVE · TRACE · SMALL · MODERATE · LARGE	HYDRATE 2AM BLOOD SUGAR _____ ADDITIONAL BLOOD SUGAR READINGS BS ___ at __ : __ AM/PM BS ___ at __ : __ AM/PM	NOTES MEDICINE

DATE: ______________________ SUN MON TUES WED THUR FRI SAT

	MEALS AND SNACKS	CARB AND FOOD CALCULATIONS	SHOT DETAILS AND LOCATION
BREAKFAST	Total Carbohydrates : ___._ grams	Correction Dose: (BS - ___) / __ (___-___)/__ = (__/__) = ___.__ Carb Dose Calculation: (Meal Carbs / ___) (__._ /___) = ___.__ Correction Dose + Carb Dose Calculation: (_____ + _____) = ___.__ OR __ UNITS Correction Dose / Dose Calculation / Rounded to nearest whole number	TIME __:__ AM / PM LEFT ARM CGM / RIGHT ARM CGM / LEFT LEG CGM / RIGHT LEG CGM / LEFT/RIGHT STOMACH CGM KETONES NEGATIVE / TRACE / SMALL / MODERATE / LARGE
SNACK	Total Carbohydrates : ___._ grams	Carb Dose Calculation: (Meal Carbs / ___) (__._ /___) = ___.__ or __ UNITS NO INSULIN DOSE REQUIRED FOR MEALS/SNACKS UNDER __G OF CARBS OR EQUAL TO __.__ OR LESS	TIME __:__ AM / PM LEFT ARM CGM / RIGHT ARM CGM / LEFT LEG CGM / RIGHT LEG CGM / LEFT/RIGHT STOMACH CGM KETONES NEGATIVE / TRACE / SMALL / MODERATE / LARGE
LUNCH	Total Carbohydrates : ___._ grams	Correction Dose: (BS - ___) / __ (___-___)/__ = (__/__) = ___.__ Carb Dose Calculation: (Meal Carbs / ___) (__._ /___) = ___.__ Correction Dose + Carb Dose Calculation: (_____ + _____) = ___.__ OR __ UNITS Correction Dose / Dose Calculation / Rounded to nearest whole number	TIME __:__ AM / PM LEFT ARM CGM / RIGHT ARM CGM / LEFT LEG CGM / RIGHT LEG CGM / LEFT/RIGHT STOMACH CGM KETONES NEGATIVE / TRACE / SMALL / MODERATE / LARGE
SNACK	Total Carbohydrates : ___._ grams	Carb Dose Calculation: (Meal Carbs / ___) (__._ /___) = ___.__ or __ UNITS NO INSULIN DOSE REQUIRED FOR MEALS/SNACKS UNDER __G OF CARBS OR EQUAL TO __.__ OR LESS	TIME __:__ AM / PM LEFT ARM CGM / RIGHT ARM CGM / LEFT LEG CGM / RIGHT LEG CGM / LEFT/RIGHT STOMACH CGM KETONES NEGATIVE / TRACE / SMALL / MODERATE / LARGE
DINNER	Total Carbohydrates : ___._ grams	Correction Dose: (BS - ___) / __ (___-___)/__ = (__/__) = ___.__ Carb Dose Calculation: (Meal Carbs / ___) (__._ /___) = ___.__ Correction Dose + Carb Dose Calculation: (_____ + _____) = ___.__ OR __ UNITS Correction Dose / Dose Calculation / Rounded to nearest whole number	TIME __:__ AM / PM LEFT ARM CGM / RIGHT ARM CGM / LEFT LEG CGM / RIGHT LEG CGM / LEFT/RIGHT STOMACH CGM KETONES NEGATIVE / TRACE / SMALL / MODERATE / LARGE
SNACK	Total Carbohydrates : ___._ grams	Carb Dose Calculation: (Meal Carbs / ___) (__._ /___) = ___.__ or __ UNITS NO INSULIN DOSE REQUIRED FOR MEALS/SNACKS UNDER __G OF CARBS OR EQUAL TO __.__ OR LESS	TIME __:__ AM / PM LEFT ARM CGM / RIGHT ARM CGM / LEFT LEG CGM / RIGHT LEG CGM / LEFT/RIGHT STOMACH CGM KETONES NEGATIVE / TRACE / SMALL / MODERATE / LARGE
BEDTIME __:__ PM	BLOOD SUGAR _____ UNITS ___ LEFT ARM CGM / RIGHT ARM CGM / LEFT LEG CGM / RIGHT LEG CGM / LEFT/RIGHT STOMACH CGM KETONES NEGATIVE / TRACE / SMALL / MODERATE / LARGE	HYDRATE 2AM BLOOD SUGAR _____ ADDITIONAL BLOOD SUGAR READINGS BS ___ at __ : __ AM/PM BS ___ at __ : __ AM/PM	NOTES MEDICINE

DATE: ______________________ SUN MON TUES WED THUR FRI SAT

	MEALS AND SNACKS	CARB AND FOOD CALCULATIONS	SHOT DETAILS AND LOCATION
BREAKFAST	Total Carbohydrates : ___._ grams	Correction Dose: (BS - ___) / __ (___-___)/__ = (__/__) = ___.__ Carb Dose Calculation: (Meal Carbs / ___) (__._ /___) = ___.__ Correction Dose + Carb Dose Calculation: (__.__ + __.__) = __.__ OR __ UNITS Correction Dose / Dose Calculation / Rounded to nearest whole number	TIME __ : __ AM / PM LEFT ARM CGM / RIGHT ARM CGM / LEFT LEG CGM / RIGHT LEG CGM / LEFT/RIGHT STOMACH CGM KETONES NEGATIVE / TRACE / SMALL / MODERATE / LARGE
SNACK	Total Carbohydrates : ___._ grams	Carb Dose Calculation: (Meal Carbs / ___) (__._ /___) = ___.__ or __ UNITS NO INSULIN DOSE REQUIRED FOR MEALS/SNACKS UNDER __G OF CARBS OR EQUAL TO __.__ OR LESS	TIME __ : __ AM / PM LEFT ARM CGM / RIGHT ARM CGM / LEFT LEG CGM / RIGHT LEG CGM / LEFT/RIGHT STOMACH CGM KETONES NEGATIVE / TRACE / SMALL / MODERATE / LARGE
LUNCH	Total Carbohydrates : ___._ grams	Correction Dose: (BS - ___) / __ (___-___)/__ = (__/__) = ___.__ Carb Dose Calculation: (Meal Carbs / ___) (__._ /___) = ___.__ Correction Dose + Carb Dose Calculation: (__.__ + __.__) = __.__ OR __ UNITS Correction Dose / Dose Calculation / Rounded to nearest whole number	TIME __ : __ AM / PM LEFT ARM CGM / RIGHT ARM CGM / LEFT LEG CGM / RIGHT LEG CGM / LEFT/RIGHT STOMACH CGM KETONES NEGATIVE / TRACE / SMALL / MODERATE / LARGE
SNACK	Total Carbohydrates : ___._ grams	Carb Dose Calculation: (Meal Carbs / ___) (__._ /___) = ___.__ or __ UNITS NO INSULIN DOSE REQUIRED FOR MEALS/SNACKS UNDER __G OF CARBS OR EQUAL TO __.__ OR LESS	TIME __ : __ AM / PM LEFT ARM CGM / RIGHT ARM CGM / LEFT LEG CGM / RIGHT LEG CGM / LEFT/RIGHT STOMACH CGM KETONES NEGATIVE / TRACE / SMALL / MODERATE / LARGE
DINNER	Total Carbohydrates : ___._ grams	Correction Dose: (BS - ___) / __ (___-___)/__ = (__/__) = ___.__ Carb Dose Calculation: (Meal Carbs / ___) (__._ /___) = ___.__ Correction Dose + Carb Dose Calculation: (__.__ + __.__) = __.__ OR __ UNITS Correction Dose / Dose Calculation / Rounded to nearest whole number	TIME __ : __ AM / PM LEFT ARM CGM / RIGHT ARM CGM / LEFT LEG CGM / RIGHT LEG CGM / LEFT/RIGHT STOMACH CGM KETONES NEGATIVE / TRACE / SMALL / MODERATE / LARGE
SNACK	Total Carbohydrates : ___._ grams	Carb Dose Calculation: (Meal Carbs / ___) (__._ /___) = ___.__ or __ UNITS NO INSULIN DOSE REQUIRED FOR MEALS/SNACKS UNDER __G OF CARBS OR EQUAL TO __.__ OR LESS	TIME __ : __ AM / PM LEFT ARM CGM / RIGHT ARM CGM / LEFT LEG CGM / RIGHT LEG CGM / LEFT/RIGHT STOMACH CGM KETONES NEGATIVE / TRACE / SMALL / MODERATE / LARGE
BEDTIME __ : __ PM	BLOOD SUGAR _____ UNITS ___ LEFT ARM CGM / RIGHT ARM CGM / LEFT LEG CGM / RIGHT LEG CGM / LEFT/RIGHT STOMACH CGM KETONES NEGATIVE / TRACE / SMALL / MODERATE / LARGE	HYDRATE 2AM BLOOD SUGAR _____ ADDITIONAL BLOOD SUGAR READINGS BS ___ at __ : __ AM/PM BS ___ at __ : __ AM/PM	NOTES MEDICINE

DATE: ______________________________ SUN MON TUES WED THUR FRI SAT

	MEALS AND SNACKS	CARB AND FOOD CALCULATIONS	SHOT DETAILS AND LOCATION
BREAKFAST	Total Carbohydrates : ___._ grams	Correction Dose: (BS - ___) / __ (___-___)/__ = (__/__) = ___.__ Carb Dose Calculation: (Meal Carbs / ___) (__._ /___) = ___.__ Correction Dose + Carb Dose Calculation: (___.__ + ___.__) = __.__ OR __ UNITS Correction Dose Dose Calculation Rounded to nearest whole number	TIME __ : __ AM / PM LEFT ARM CGM | RIGHT ARM CGM | LEFT LEG CGM | RIGHT LEG CGM | LEFT/RIGHT STOMACH CGM KETONES NEGATIVE TRACE SMALL MODERATE LARGE
SNACK	Total Carbohydrates : ___._ grams	Carb Dose Calculation: (Meal Carbs / ___) (__._ /___) = ___.__ or __ UNITS NO INSULIN DOSE REQUIRED FOR MEALS/SNACKS UNDER __G OF CARBS OR EQUAL TO __.__ OR LESS	TIME __ : __ AM / PM LEFT ARM CGM | RIGHT ARM CGM | LEFT LEG CGM | RIGHT LEG CGM | LEFT/RIGHT STOMACH CGM KETONES NEGATIVE TRACE SMALL MODERATE LARGE
LUNCH	Total Carbohydrates : ___._ grams	Correction Dose: (BS - ___) / __ (___-___)/__ = (__/__) = ___.__ Carb Dose Calculation: (Meal Carbs / ___) (__._ /___) = ___.__ Correction Dose + Carb Dose Calculation: (___.__ + ___.__) = __.__ OR __ UNITS Correction Dose Dose Calculation Rounded to nearest whole number	TIME __ : __ AM / PM LEFT ARM CGM | RIGHT ARM CGM | LEFT LEG CGM | RIGHT LEG CGM | LEFT/RIGHT STOMACH CGM KETONES NEGATIVE TRACE SMALL MODERATE LARGE
SNACK	Total Carbohydrates : ___._ grams	Carb Dose Calculation: (Meal Carbs / ___) (__._ /___) = ___.__ or __ UNITS NO INSULIN DOSE REQUIRED FOR MEALS/SNACKS UNDER __G OF CARBS OR EQUAL TO __.__ OR LESS	TIME __ : __ AM / PM LEFT ARM CGM | RIGHT ARM CGM | LEFT LEG CGM | RIGHT LEG CGM | LEFT/RIGHT STOMACH CGM KETONES NEGATIVE TRACE SMALL MODERATE LARGE
DINNER	Total Carbohydrates : ___._ grams	Correction Dose: (BS - ___) / __ (___-___)/__ = (__/__) = ___.__ Carb Dose Calculation: (Meal Carbs / ___) (__._ /___) = ___.__ Correction Dose + Carb Dose Calculation: (___.__ + ___.__) = __.__ OR __ UNITS Correction Dose Dose Calculation Rounded to nearest whole number	TIME __ : __ AM / PM LEFT ARM CGM | RIGHT ARM CGM | LEFT LEG CGM | RIGHT LEG CGM | LEFT/RIGHT STOMACH CGM KETONES NEGATIVE TRACE SMALL MODERATE LARGE
SNACK	Total Carbohydrates : ___._ grams	Carb Dose Calculation: (Meal Carbs / ___) (__._ /___) = ___.__ or __ UNITS NO INSULIN DOSE REQUIRED FOR MEALS/SNACKS UNDER __G OF CARBS OR EQUAL TO __.__ OR LESS	TIME __ : __ AM / PM LEFT ARM CGM | RIGHT ARM CGM | LEFT LEG CGM | RIGHT LEG CGM | LEFT/RIGHT STOMACH CGM KETONES NEGATIVE TRACE SMALL MODERATE LARGE
BEDTIME __ : __ PM	BLOOD SUGAR _____ UNITS ___ LEFT ARM CGM | RIGHT ARM CGM | LEFT LEG CGM | RIGHT LEG CGM | LEFT/RIGHT STOMACH CGM KETONES NEGATIVE TRACE SMALL MODERATE LARGE	HYDRATE 2AM BLOOD SUGAR _____ ADDITIONAL BLOOD SUGAR READINGS BS ___ at __ : __ AM/PM BS ___ at __ : __ AM/PM	NOTES MEDICINE

DATE: ______________________ SUN MON TUES WED THUR FRI SAT

	MEALS AND SNACKS	CARB AND FOOD CALCULATIONS	SHOT DETAILS AND LOCATION
BREAKFAST	Total Carbohydrates : ___._ grams	Correction Dose: (BS - ___) / __ (___-___)/__ = (__/__) = ___.__ Carb Dose Calculation: (Meal Carbs / ___) (__._ /___) = ___.__ Correction Dose + Carb Dose Calculation: (______ + ______) = __.__ OR __ UNITS Correction Dose, Dose Calculation, Rounded to nearest whole number	TIME __ : __ AM / PM LEFT ARM CGM / RIGHT ARM CGM / LEFT LEG CGM / RIGHT LEG CGM / LEFT/RIGHT STOMACH CGM KETONES NEGATIVE TRACE SMALL MODERATE LARGE
SNACK	Total Carbohydrates : ___._ grams	Carb Dose Calculation: (Meal Carbs / ___) (__._ /___) = ___.__ or __ UNITS NO INSULIN DOSE REQUIRED FOR MEALS/SNACKS UNDER __G OF CARBS OR EQUAL TO __.__ OR LESS	TIME __ : __ AM / PM LEFT ARM CGM / RIGHT ARM CGM / LEFT LEG CGM / RIGHT LEG CGM / LEFT/RIGHT STOMACH CGM KETONES NEGATIVE TRACE SMALL MODERATE LARGE
LUNCH	Total Carbohydrates : ___._ grams	Correction Dose: (BS - ___) / __ (___-___)/__ = (__/__) = ___.__ Carb Dose Calculation: (Meal Carbs / ___) (__._ /___) = ___.__ Correction Dose + Carb Dose Calculation: (______ + ______) = __.__ OR __ UNITS Correction Dose, Dose Calculation, Rounded to nearest whole number	TIME __ : __ AM / PM LEFT ARM CGM / RIGHT ARM CGM / LEFT LEG CGM / RIGHT LEG CGM / LEFT/RIGHT STOMACH CGM KETONES NEGATIVE TRACE SMALL MODERATE LARGE
SNACK	Total Carbohydrates : ___._ grams	Carb Dose Calculation: (Meal Carbs / ___) (__._ /___) = ___.__ or __ UNITS NO INSULIN DOSE REQUIRED FOR MEALS/SNACKS UNDER __G OF CARBS OR EQUAL TO __.__ OR LESS	TIME __ : __ AM / PM LEFT ARM CGM / RIGHT ARM CGM / LEFT LEG CGM / RIGHT LEG CGM / LEFT/RIGHT STOMACH CGM KETONES NEGATIVE TRACE SMALL MODERATE LARGE
DINNER	Total Carbohydrates : ___._ grams	Correction Dose: (BS - ___) / __ (___-___)/__ = (__/__) = ___.__ Carb Dose Calculation: (Meal Carbs / ___) (__._ /___) = ___.__ Correction Dose + Carb Dose Calculation: (______ + ______) = __.__ OR __ UNITS Correction Dose, Dose Calculation, Rounded to nearest whole number	TIME __ : __ AM / PM LEFT ARM CGM / RIGHT ARM CGM / LEFT LEG CGM / RIGHT LEG CGM / LEFT/RIGHT STOMACH CGM KETONES NEGATIVE TRACE SMALL MODERATE LARGE
SNACK	Total Carbohydrates : ___._ grams	Carb Dose Calculation: (Meal Carbs / ___) (__._ /___) = ___.__ or __ UNITS NO INSULIN DOSE REQUIRED FOR MEALS/SNACKS UNDER __G OF CARBS OR EQUAL TO __.__ OR LESS	TIME __ : __ AM / PM LEFT ARM CGM / RIGHT ARM CGM / LEFT LEG CGM / RIGHT LEG CGM / LEFT/RIGHT STOMACH CGM KETONES NEGATIVE TRACE SMALL MODERATE LARGE
BEDTIME __ : __ PM	BLOOD SUGAR _____ UNITS ___ LEFT ARM CGM / RIGHT ARM CGM / LEFT LEG CGM / RIGHT LEG CGM / LEFT/RIGHT STOMACH CGM KETONES NEGATIVE TRACE SMALL MODERATE LARGE	HYDRATE 2AM BLOOD SUGAR _____ ADDITIONAL BLOOD SUGAR READINGS BS ___ at __ : __ AM/PM BS ___ at __ : __ AM/PM	NOTES MEDICINE

DATE: ______________________ SUN MON TUES WED THUR FRI SAT

	MEALS AND SNACKS	CARB AND FOOD CALCULATIONS	SHOT DETAILS AND LOCATION
BREAKFAST	Total Carbohydrates : ___._ grams	Correction Dose: (BS - ___) / __ (___-___)/__ = (__/__) = ___.__ Carb Dose Calculation: (Meal Carbs / ___) (__._ /___) = ___.__ Correction Dose + Carb Dose Calculation: (_____ + _____) = __.__ OR __ UNITS Correction Dose / Dose Calculation / Rounded to nearest whole number	TIME __ : __ AM / PM LEFT ARM CGM / RIGHT ARM CGM / LEFT LEG CGM / RIGHT LEG CGM / LEFT/RIGHT STOMACH CGM KETONES NEGATIVE / TRACE / SMALL / MODERATE / LARGE
SNACK	Total Carbohydrates : ___._ grams	Carb Dose Calculation: (Meal Carbs / ___) (__._ /___) = ___.__ or __ UNITS NO INSULIN DOSE REQUIRED FOR MEALS/SNACKS UNDER __G OF CARBS OR EQUAL TO __.__ OR LESS	TIME __ : __ AM / PM LEFT ARM CGM / RIGHT ARM CGM / LEFT LEG CGM / RIGHT LEG CGM / LEFT/RIGHT STOMACH CGM KETONES NEGATIVE / TRACE / SMALL / MODERATE / LARGE
LUNCH	Total Carbohydrates : ___._ grams	Correction Dose: (BS - ___) / __ (___-___)/__ = (__/__) = ___.__ Carb Dose Calculation: (Meal Carbs / ___) (__._ /___) = ___.__ Correction Dose + Carb Dose Calculation: (_____ + _____) = __.__ OR __ UNITS Correction Dose / Dose Calculation / Rounded to nearest whole number	TIME __ : __ AM / PM LEFT ARM CGM / RIGHT ARM CGM / LEFT LEG CGM / RIGHT LEG CGM / LEFT/RIGHT STOMACH CGM KETONES NEGATIVE / TRACE / SMALL / MODERATE / LARGE
SNACK	Total Carbohydrates : ___._ grams	Carb Dose Calculation: (Meal Carbs / ___) (__._ /___) = ___.__ or __ UNITS NO INSULIN DOSE REQUIRED FOR MEALS/SNACKS UNDER __G OF CARBS OR EQUAL TO __.__ OR LESS	TIME __ : __ AM / PM LEFT ARM CGM / RIGHT ARM CGM / LEFT LEG CGM / RIGHT LEG CGM / LEFT/RIGHT STOMACH CGM KETONES NEGATIVE / TRACE / SMALL / MODERATE / LARGE
DINNER	Total Carbohydrates : ___._ grams	Correction Dose: (BS - ___) / __ (___-___)/__ = (__/__) = ___.__ Carb Dose Calculation: (Meal Carbs / ___) (__._ /___) = ___.__ Correction Dose + Carb Dose Calculation: (_____ + _____) = __.__ OR __ UNITS Correction Dose / Dose Calculation / Rounded to nearest whole number	TIME __ : __ AM / PM LEFT ARM CGM / RIGHT ARM CGM / LEFT LEG CGM / RIGHT LEG CGM / LEFT/RIGHT STOMACH CGM KETONES NEGATIVE / TRACE / SMALL / MODERATE / LARGE
SNACK	Total Carbohydrates : ___._ grams	Carb Dose Calculation: (Meal Carbs / ___) (__._ /___) = ___.__ or __ UNITS NO INSULIN DOSE REQUIRED FOR MEALS/SNACKS UNDER __G OF CARBS OR EQUAL TO __.__ OR LESS	TIME __ : __ AM / PM LEFT ARM CGM / RIGHT ARM CGM / LEFT LEG CGM / RIGHT LEG CGM / LEFT/RIGHT STOMACH CGM KETONES NEGATIVE / TRACE / SMALL / MODERATE / LARGE
BEDTIME __ : __ PM	BLOOD SUGAR _____ UNITS ___ LEFT ARM CGM / RIGHT ARM CGM / LEFT LEG CGM / RIGHT LEG CGM / LEFT/RIGHT STOMACH CGM KETONES NEGATIVE / TRACE / SMALL / MODERATE / LARGE	HYDRATE 2AM BLOOD SUGAR _____ ADDITIONAL BLOOD SUGAR READINGS BS ___ at __ : __ AM/PM BS ___ at __ : __ AM/PM	NOTES MEDICINE

DATE: ______________________________ SUN MON TUES WED THUR FRI SAT

	MEALS AND SNACKS	CARB AND FOOD CALCULATIONS	SHOT DETAILS AND LOCATION
BREAKFAST	Total Carbohydrates : ___._ grams	Correction Dose: (BS - ___) / __ (___-___)/__ = (__/__) = ___.__ Carb Dose Calculation: (Meal Carbs / ___) (__._ /___) = ___.__ Correction Dose + Carb Dose Calculation: (__.__ + __.__) = __.__ OR __ UNITS Correction Dose, Dose Calculation, Rounded to nearest whole number	TIME __ : __ AM / PM LEFT ARM CGM, RIGHT ARM CGM, LEFT LEG CGM, RIGHT LEG CGM, LEFT/RIGHT STOMACH CGM KETONES NEGATIVE, TRACE, SMALL, MODERATE, LARGE
SNACK	Total Carbohydrates : ___._ grams	Carb Dose Calculation: (Meal Carbs / ___) (__._ /___) = ___.__ or __ UNITS NO INSULIN DOSE REQUIRED FOR MEALS/SNACKS UNDER __G OF CARBS OR EQUAL TO __.__ OR LESS	TIME __ : __ AM / PM LEFT ARM CGM, RIGHT ARM CGM, LEFT LEG CGM, RIGHT LEG CGM, LEFT/RIGHT STOMACH CGM KETONES NEGATIVE, TRACE, SMALL, MODERATE, LARGE
LUNCH	Total Carbohydrates : ___._ grams	Correction Dose: (BS - ___) / __ (___-___)/__ = (__/__) = ___.__ Carb Dose Calculation: (Meal Carbs / ___) (__._ /___) = ___.__ Correction Dose + Carb Dose Calculation: (__.__ + __.__) = __.__ OR __ UNITS Correction Dose, Dose Calculation, Rounded to nearest whole number	TIME __ : __ AM / PM LEFT ARM CGM, RIGHT ARM CGM, LEFT LEG CGM, RIGHT LEG CGM, LEFT/RIGHT STOMACH CGM KETONES NEGATIVE, TRACE, SMALL, MODERATE, LARGE
SNACK	Total Carbohydrates : ___._ grams	Carb Dose Calculation: (Meal Carbs / ___) (__._ /___) = ___.__ or __ UNITS NO INSULIN DOSE REQUIRED FOR MEALS/SNACKS UNDER __G OF CARBS OR EQUAL TO __.__ OR LESS	TIME __ : __ AM / PM LEFT ARM CGM, RIGHT ARM CGM, LEFT LEG CGM, RIGHT LEG CGM, LEFT/RIGHT STOMACH CGM KETONES NEGATIVE, TRACE, SMALL, MODERATE, LARGE
DINNER	Total Carbohydrates : ___._ grams	Correction Dose: (BS - ___) / __ (___-___)/__ = (__/__) = ___.__ Carb Dose Calculation: (Meal Carbs / ___) (__._ /___) = ___.__ Correction Dose + Carb Dose Calculation: (__.__ + __.__) = __.__ OR __ UNITS Correction Dose, Dose Calculation, Rounded to nearest whole number	TIME __ : __ AM / PM LEFT ARM CGM, RIGHT ARM CGM, LEFT LEG CGM, RIGHT LEG CGM, LEFT/RIGHT STOMACH CGM KETONES NEGATIVE, TRACE, SMALL, MODERATE, LARGE
SNACK	Total Carbohydrates : ___._ grams	Carb Dose Calculation: (Meal Carbs / ___) (__._ /___) = ___.__ or __ UNITS NO INSULIN DOSE REQUIRED FOR MEALS/SNACKS UNDER __G OF CARBS OR EQUAL TO __.__ OR LESS	TIME __ : __ AM / PM LEFT ARM CGM, RIGHT ARM CGM, LEFT LEG CGM, RIGHT LEG CGM, LEFT/RIGHT STOMACH CGM KETONES NEGATIVE, TRACE, SMALL, MODERATE, LARGE
BEDTIME __ : __ PM	BLOOD SUGAR _____ UNITS ___ LEFT ARM CGM, RIGHT ARM CGM, LEFT LEG CGM, RIGHT LEG CGM, LEFT/RIGHT STOMACH CGM KETONES NEGATIVE, TRACE, SMALL, MODERATE, LARGE	HYDRATE 2AM BLOOD SUGAR _____ ADDITIONAL BLOOD SUGAR READINGS BS ___ at __ : __ AM/PM BS ___ at __ : __ AM/PM	NOTES MEDICINE

DATE: ______________________ SUN MON TUES WED THUR FRI SAT

	MEALS AND SNACKS	CARB AND FOOD CALCULATIONS	SHOT DETAILS AND LOCATION
BREAKFAST	Total Carbohydrates : ___._ grams	Correction Dose: (BS - ___) / __ (___-___)/__ = (__/__) = ___.__ Carb Dose Calculation: (Meal Carbs / ___) (__._ /___) = ___.__ Correction Dose + Carb Dose Calculation: (_____ + _____) = ___.__ OR __ UNITS Correction Dose Dose Calculation Rounded to nearest whole number	TIME __ : __ AM / PM LEFT ARM CGM · RIGHT ARM CGM · LEFT LEG CGM · RIGHT LEG CGM · LEFT/RIGHT STOMACH CGM KETONES NEGATIVE TRACE SMALL MODERATE LARGE
SNACK	Total Carbohydrates : ___._ grams	Carb Dose Calculation: (Meal Carbs / ___) (__._ /___) = ___.__ or __ UNITS NO INSULIN DOSE REQUIRED FOR MEALS/SNACKS UNDER __G OF CARBS OR EQUAL TO __.__ OR LESS	TIME __ : __ AM / PM LEFT ARM CGM · RIGHT ARM CGM · LEFT LEG CGM · RIGHT LEG CGM · LEFT/RIGHT STOMACH CGM KETONES NEGATIVE TRACE SMALL MODERATE LARGE
LUNCH	Total Carbohydrates : ___._ grams	Correction Dose: (BS - ___) / __ (___-___)/__ = (__/__) = ___.__ Carb Dose Calculation: (Meal Carbs / ___) (__._ /___) = ___.__ Correction Dose + Carb Dose Calculation: (_____ + _____) = ___.__ OR __ UNITS Correction Dose Dose Calculation Rounded to nearest whole number	TIME __ : __ AM / PM LEFT ARM CGM · RIGHT ARM CGM · LEFT LEG CGM · RIGHT LEG CGM · LEFT/RIGHT STOMACH CGM KETONES NEGATIVE TRACE SMALL MODERATE LARGE
SNACK	Total Carbohydrates : ___._ grams	Carb Dose Calculation: (Meal Carbs / ___) (__._ /___) = ___.__ or __ UNITS NO INSULIN DOSE REQUIRED FOR MEALS/SNACKS UNDER __G OF CARBS OR EQUAL TO __.__ OR LESS	TIME __ : __ AM / PM LEFT ARM CGM · RIGHT ARM CGM · LEFT LEG CGM · RIGHT LEG CGM · LEFT/RIGHT STOMACH CGM KETONES NEGATIVE TRACE SMALL MODERATE LARGE
DINNER	Total Carbohydrates : ___._ grams	Correction Dose: (BS - ___) / __ (___-___)/__ = (__/__) = ___.__ Carb Dose Calculation: (Meal Carbs / ___) (__._ /___) = ___.__ Correction Dose + Carb Dose Calculation: (_____ + _____) = ___.__ OR __ UNITS Correction Dose Dose Calculation Rounded to nearest whole number	TIME __ : __ AM / PM LEFT ARM CGM · RIGHT ARM CGM · LEFT LEG CGM · RIGHT LEG CGM · LEFT/RIGHT STOMACH CGM KETONES NEGATIVE TRACE SMALL MODERATE LARGE
SNACK	Total Carbohydrates : ___._ grams	Carb Dose Calculation: (Meal Carbs / ___) (__._ /___) = ___.__ or __ UNITS NO INSULIN DOSE REQUIRED FOR MEALS/SNACKS UNDER __G OF CARBS OR EQUAL TO __.__ OR LESS	TIME __ : __ AM / PM LEFT ARM CGM · RIGHT ARM CGM · LEFT LEG CGM · RIGHT LEG CGM · LEFT/RIGHT STOMACH CGM KETONES NEGATIVE TRACE SMALL MODERATE LARGE
BEDTIME __ : __ PM	BLOOD SUGAR _____ UNITS ___ LEFT ARM CGM · RIGHT ARM CGM · LEFT LEG CGM · RIGHT LEG CGM · LEFT/RIGHT STOMACH CGM KETONES NEGATIVE TRACE SMALL MODERATE LARGE	HYDRATE 2AM BLOOD SUGAR _____ ADDITIONAL BLOOD SUGAR READINGS BS ___ at __ : __ AM/PM BS ___ at __ : __ AM/PM	NOTES MEDICINE

DATE: ______________________________ SUN MON TUES WED THUR FRI SAT

	MEALS AND SNACKS	CARB AND FOOD CALCULATIONS	SHOT DETAILS AND LOCATION
BREAKFAST	Total Carbohydrates : ___._ grams	Correction Dose: (BS - ___) / __ (___-___)/__ = (__/__) = ___.__ Carb Dose Calculation: (Meal Carbs / ___) (__._ /___) = ___.__ Correction Dose + Carb Dose Calculation: (_____ + _____) = __.__ OR __ UNITS Correction Dose / Dose Calculation / Rounded to nearest whole number	TIME __:__ AM / PM LEFT ARM CGM / RIGHT ARM CGM / LEFT LEG CGM / RIGHT LEG CGM / LEFT/RIGHT STOMACH CGM KETONES NEGATIVE TRACE SMALL MODERATE LARGE
SNACK	Total Carbohydrates : ___._ grams	Carb Dose Calculation: (Meal Carbs / ___) (__._ /___) = ___.__ or __ UNITS NO INSULIN DOSE REQUIRED FOR MEALS/SNACKS UNDER __G OF CARBS OR EQUAL TO __.__ OR LESS	TIME __:__ AM / PM LEFT ARM CGM / RIGHT ARM CGM / LEFT LEG CGM / RIGHT LEG CGM / LEFT/RIGHT STOMACH CGM KETONES NEGATIVE TRACE SMALL MODERATE LARGE
LUNCH	Total Carbohydrates : ___._ grams	Correction Dose: (BS - ___) / __ (___-___)/__ = (__/__) = ___.__ Carb Dose Calculation: (Meal Carbs / ___) (__._ /___) = ___.__ Correction Dose + Carb Dose Calculation: (_____ + _____) = __.__ OR __ UNITS Correction Dose / Dose Calculation / Rounded to nearest whole number	TIME __:__ AM / PM LEFT ARM CGM / RIGHT ARM CGM / LEFT LEG CGM / RIGHT LEG CGM / LEFT/RIGHT STOMACH CGM KETONES NEGATIVE TRACE SMALL MODERATE LARGE
SNACK	Total Carbohydrates : ___._ grams	Carb Dose Calculation: (Meal Carbs / ___) (__._ /___) = ___.__ or __ UNITS NO INSULIN DOSE REQUIRED FOR MEALS/SNACKS UNDER __G OF CARBS OR EQUAL TO __.__ OR LESS	TIME __:__ AM / PM LEFT ARM CGM / RIGHT ARM CGM / LEFT LEG CGM / RIGHT LEG CGM / LEFT/RIGHT STOMACH CGM KETONES NEGATIVE TRACE SMALL MODERATE LARGE
DINNER	Total Carbohydrates : ___._ grams	Correction Dose: (BS - ___) / __ (___-___)/__ = (__/__) = ___.__ Carb Dose Calculation: (Meal Carbs / ___) (__._ /___) = ___.__ Correction Dose + Carb Dose Calculation: (_____ + _____) = __.__ OR __ UNITS Correction Dose / Dose Calculation / Rounded to nearest whole number	TIME __:__ AM / PM LEFT ARM CGM / RIGHT ARM CGM / LEFT LEG CGM / RIGHT LEG CGM / LEFT/RIGHT STOMACH CGM KETONES NEGATIVE TRACE SMALL MODERATE LARGE
SNACK	Total Carbohydrates : ___._ grams	Carb Dose Calculation: (Meal Carbs / ___) (__._ /___) = ___.__ or __ UNITS NO INSULIN DOSE REQUIRED FOR MEALS/SNACKS UNDER __G OF CARBS OR EQUAL TO __.__ OR LESS	TIME __:__ AM / PM LEFT ARM CGM / RIGHT ARM CGM / LEFT LEG CGM / RIGHT LEG CGM / LEFT/RIGHT STOMACH CGM KETONES NEGATIVE TRACE SMALL MODERATE LARGE
BEDTIME __:__ PM	BLOOD SUGAR _____ UNITS ___ LEFT ARM CGM / RIGHT ARM CGM / LEFT LEG CGM / RIGHT LEG CGM / LEFT/RIGHT STOMACH CGM KETONES NEGATIVE TRACE SMALL MODERATE LARGE	HYDRATE 2AM BLOOD SUGAR _____ ADDITIONAL BLOOD SUGAR READINGS BS ___ at __ : __ AM/PM BS ___ at __ : __ AM/PM	NOTES MEDICINE

DATE: ____________________ SUN MON TUES WED THUR FRI SAT

	MEALS AND SNACKS	CARB AND FOOD CALCULATIONS	SHOT DETAILS AND LOCATION
BREAKFAST	Total Carbohydrates : ___._ grams	Correction Dose: (BS - ___) / __ (___-___)/__ = (__/__) = ___.__ Carb Dose Calculation: (Meal Carbs / ___) (__._ /___) = ___.__ Correction Dose + Carb Dose Calculation: (__.__ + __.__) = __.__ OR __ UNITS Correction Dose · Dose Calculation · Rounded to nearest whole number	TIME __ : __ AM / PM LEFT ARM CGM · RIGHT ARM CGM · LEFT LEG CGM · RIGHT LEG CGM · LEFT/RIGHT STOMACH CGM KETONES NEGATIVE · TRACE · SMALL · MODERATE · LARGE
SNACK	Total Carbohydrates : ___._ grams	Carb Dose Calculation: (Meal Carbs / ___) (__._ /___) = ___.__ or __ UNITS NO INSULIN DOSE REQUIRED FOR MEALS/SNACKS UNDER __G OF CARBS OR EQUAL TO __.__ OR LESS	TIME __ : __ AM / PM LEFT ARM CGM · RIGHT ARM CGM · LEFT LEG CGM · RIGHT LEG CGM · LEFT/RIGHT STOMACH CGM KETONES NEGATIVE · TRACE · SMALL · MODERATE · LARGE
LUNCH	Total Carbohydrates : ___._ grams	Correction Dose: (BS - ___) / __ (___-___)/__ = (__/__) = ___.__ Carb Dose Calculation: (Meal Carbs / ___) (__._ /___) = ___.__ Correction Dose + Carb Dose Calculation: (__.__ + __.__) = __.__ OR __ UNITS Correction Dose · Dose Calculation · Rounded to nearest whole number	TIME __ : __ AM / PM LEFT ARM CGM · RIGHT ARM CGM · LEFT LEG CGM · RIGHT LEG CGM · LEFT/RIGHT STOMACH CGM KETONES NEGATIVE · TRACE · SMALL · MODERATE · LARGE
SNACK	Total Carbohydrates : ___._ grams	Carb Dose Calculation: (Meal Carbs / ___) (__._ /___) = ___.__ or __ UNITS NO INSULIN DOSE REQUIRED FOR MEALS/SNACKS UNDER __G OF CARBS OR EQUAL TO __.__ OR LESS	TIME __ : __ AM / PM LEFT ARM CGM · RIGHT ARM CGM · LEFT LEG CGM · RIGHT LEG CGM · LEFT/RIGHT STOMACH CGM KETONES NEGATIVE · TRACE · SMALL · MODERATE · LARGE
DINNER	Total Carbohydrates : ___._ grams	Correction Dose: (BS - ___) / __ (___-___)/__ = (__/__) = ___.__ Carb Dose Calculation: (Meal Carbs / ___) (__._ /___) = ___.__ Correction Dose + Carb Dose Calculation: (__.__ + __.__) = __.__ OR __ UNITS Correction Dose · Dose Calculation · Rounded to nearest whole number	TIME __ : __ AM / PM LEFT ARM CGM · RIGHT ARM CGM · LEFT LEG CGM · RIGHT LEG CGM · LEFT/RIGHT STOMACH CGM KETONES NEGATIVE · TRACE · SMALL · MODERATE · LARGE
SNACK	Total Carbohydrates : ___._ grams	Carb Dose Calculation: (Meal Carbs / ___) (__._ /___) = ___.__ or __ UNITS NO INSULIN DOSE REQUIRED FOR MEALS/SNACKS UNDER __G OF CARBS OR EQUAL TO __.__ OR LESS	TIME __ : __ AM / PM LEFT ARM CGM · RIGHT ARM CGM · LEFT LEG CGM · RIGHT LEG CGM · LEFT/RIGHT STOMACH CGM KETONES NEGATIVE · TRACE · SMALL · MODERATE · LARGE
BEDTIME __ : __ PM	BLOOD SUGAR _____ UNITS ___ LEFT ARM CGM · RIGHT ARM CGM · LEFT LEG CGM · RIGHT LEG CGM · LEFT/RIGHT STOMACH CGM KETONES NEGATIVE · TRACE · SMALL · MODERATE · LARGE	HYDRATE 2AM BLOOD SUGAR _____ ADDITIONAL BLOOD SUGAR READINGS BS ___ at __ : __ AM/PM BS ___ at __ : __ AM/PM	NOTES MEDICINE

DATE: ____________________ SUN MON TUES WED THUR FRI SAT

	MEALS AND SNACKS	CARB AND FOOD CALCULATIONS	SHOT DETAILS AND LOCATION
BREAKFAST	Total Carbohydrates : ___._ grams	Correction Dose: (BS - ___) / __ (___-___)/__ = (__/__) = ___.__ Carb Dose Calculation: (Meal Carbs / ___) (__._ /___) = ___.__ Correction Dose + Carb Dose Calculation: (__.__ + __.__) = __.__ OR __ UNITS Correction Dose / Dose Calculation / Rounded to nearest whole number	TIME __ : __ AM / PM LEFT ARM CGM / RIGHT ARM CGM / LEFT LEG CGM / RIGHT LEG CGM / LEFT/RIGHT STOMACH CGM KETONES NEGATIVE / TRACE / SMALL / MODERATE / LARGE
SNACK	Total Carbohydrates : ___._ grams	Carb Dose Calculation: (Meal Carbs / ___) (__._ /___) = ___.__ or __ UNITS NO INSULIN DOSE REQUIRED FOR MEALS/SNACKS UNDER __G OF CARBS OR EQUAL TO __.__ OR LESS	TIME __ : __ AM / PM LEFT ARM CGM / RIGHT ARM CGM / LEFT LEG CGM / RIGHT LEG CGM / LEFT/RIGHT STOMACH CGM KETONES NEGATIVE / TRACE / SMALL / MODERATE / LARGE
LUNCH	Total Carbohydrates : ___._ grams	Correction Dose: (BS - ___) / __ (___-___)/__ = (__/__) = ___.__ Carb Dose Calculation: (Meal Carbs / ___) (__._ /___) = ___.__ Correction Dose + Carb Dose Calculation: (__.__ + __.__) = __.__ OR __ UNITS Correction Dose / Dose Calculation / Rounded to nearest whole number	TIME __ : __ AM / PM LEFT ARM CGM / RIGHT ARM CGM / LEFT LEG CGM / RIGHT LEG CGM / LEFT/RIGHT STOMACH CGM KETONES NEGATIVE / TRACE / SMALL / MODERATE / LARGE
SNACK	Total Carbohydrates : ___._ grams	Carb Dose Calculation: (Meal Carbs / ___) (__._ /___) = ___.__ or __ UNITS NO INSULIN DOSE REQUIRED FOR MEALS/SNACKS UNDER __G OF CARBS OR EQUAL TO __.__ OR LESS	TIME __ : __ AM / PM LEFT ARM CGM / RIGHT ARM CGM / LEFT LEG CGM / RIGHT LEG CGM / LEFT/RIGHT STOMACH CGM KETONES NEGATIVE / TRACE / SMALL / MODERATE / LARGE
DINNER	Total Carbohydrates : ___._ grams	Correction Dose: (BS - ___) / __ (___-___)/__ = (__/__) = ___.__ Carb Dose Calculation: (Meal Carbs / ___) (__._ /___) = ___.__ Correction Dose + Carb Dose Calculation: (__.__ + __.__) = __.__ OR __ UNITS Correction Dose / Dose Calculation / Rounded to nearest whole number	TIME __ : __ AM / PM LEFT ARM CGM / RIGHT ARM CGM / LEFT LEG CGM / RIGHT LEG CGM / LEFT/RIGHT STOMACH CGM KETONES NEGATIVE / TRACE / SMALL / MODERATE / LARGE
SNACK	Total Carbohydrates : ___._ grams	Carb Dose Calculation: (Meal Carbs / ___) (__._ /___) = ___.__ or __ UNITS NO INSULIN DOSE REQUIRED FOR MEALS/SNACKS UNDER __G OF CARBS OR EQUAL TO __.__ OR LESS	TIME __ : __ AM / PM LEFT ARM CGM / RIGHT ARM CGM / LEFT LEG CGM / RIGHT LEG CGM / LEFT/RIGHT STOMACH CGM KETONES NEGATIVE / TRACE / SMALL / MODERATE / LARGE
BEDTIME __ : __ PM	BLOOD SUGAR _____ UNITS ___ LEFT ARM CGM / RIGHT ARM CGM / LEFT LEG CGM / RIGHT LEG CGM / LEFT/RIGHT STOMACH CGM KETONES NEGATIVE / TRACE / SMALL / MODERATE / LARGE	HYDRATE 2AM BLOOD SUGAR _____ ADDITIONAL BLOOD SUGAR READINGS BS ___ at __ : __ AM/PM BS ___ at __ : __ AM/PM	NOTES MEDICINE

DATE: ______________________________ SUN MON TUES WED THUR FRI SAT

	MEALS AND SNACKS	CARB AND FOOD CALCULATIONS	SHOT DETAILS AND LOCATION
BREAKFAST	Total Carbohydrates : ___._ grams	Correction Dose: (BS - ___) / __ (___-___)/__ = (__/__) = ___.__ Carb Dose Calculation: (Meal Carbs / ___) (__._ /___) = ___.__ Correction Dose + Carb Dose Calculation: (__.__ + __.__) = __.__ OR __ UNITS Correction Dose, Dose Calculation, Rounded to nearest whole number	TIME __ : __ AM / PM LEFT ARM CGM, RIGHT ARM CGM, LEFT LEG CGM, RIGHT LEG CGM, LEFT/RIGHT STOMACH CGM KETONES NEGATIVE, TRACE, SMALL, MODERATE, LARGE
SNACK	Total Carbohydrates : ___._ grams	Carb Dose Calculation: (Meal Carbs / ___) (__._ /___) = ___.__ or __ UNITS NO INSULIN DOSE REQUIRED FOR MEALS/SNACKS UNDER __G OF CARBS OR EQUAL TO __.__ OR LESS	TIME __ : __ AM / PM LEFT ARM CGM, RIGHT ARM CGM, LEFT LEG CGM, RIGHT LEG CGM, LEFT/RIGHT STOMACH CGM KETONES NEGATIVE, TRACE, SMALL, MODERATE, LARGE
LUNCH	Total Carbohydrates : ___._ grams	Correction Dose: (BS - ___) / __ (___-___)/__ = (__/__) = ___.__ Carb Dose Calculation: (Meal Carbs / ___) (__._ /___) = ___.__ Correction Dose + Carb Dose Calculation: (__.__ + __.__) = __.__ OR __ UNITS Correction Dose, Dose Calculation, Rounded to nearest whole number	TIME __ : __ AM / PM LEFT ARM CGM, RIGHT ARM CGM, LEFT LEG CGM, RIGHT LEG CGM, LEFT/RIGHT STOMACH CGM KETONES NEGATIVE, TRACE, SMALL, MODERATE, LARGE
SNACK	Total Carbohydrates : ___._ grams	Carb Dose Calculation: (Meal Carbs / ___) (__._ /___) = ___.__ or __ UNITS NO INSULIN DOSE REQUIRED FOR MEALS/SNACKS UNDER __G OF CARBS OR EQUAL TO __.__ OR LESS	TIME __ : __ AM / PM LEFT ARM CGM, RIGHT ARM CGM, LEFT LEG CGM, RIGHT LEG CGM, LEFT/RIGHT STOMACH CGM KETONES NEGATIVE, TRACE, SMALL, MODERATE, LARGE
DINNER	Total Carbohydrates : ___._ grams	Correction Dose: (BS - ___) / __ (___-___)/__ = (__/__) = ___.__ Carb Dose Calculation: (Meal Carbs / ___) (__._ /___) = ___.__ Correction Dose + Carb Dose Calculation: (__.__ + __.__) = __.__ OR __ UNITS Correction Dose, Dose Calculation, Rounded to nearest whole number	TIME __ : __ AM / PM LEFT ARM CGM, RIGHT ARM CGM, LEFT LEG CGM, RIGHT LEG CGM, LEFT/RIGHT STOMACH CGM KETONES NEGATIVE, TRACE, SMALL, MODERATE, LARGE
SNACK	Total Carbohydrates : ___._ grams	Carb Dose Calculation: (Meal Carbs / ___) (__._ /___) = ___.__ or __ UNITS NO INSULIN DOSE REQUIRED FOR MEALS/SNACKS UNDER __G OF CARBS OR EQUAL TO __.__ OR LESS	TIME __ : __ AM / PM LEFT ARM CGM, RIGHT ARM CGM, LEFT LEG CGM, RIGHT LEG CGM, LEFT/RIGHT STOMACH CGM KETONES NEGATIVE, TRACE, SMALL, MODERATE, LARGE
BEDTIME __ : __ PM	BLOOD SUGAR _____ UNITS ___ LEFT ARM CGM, RIGHT ARM CGM, LEFT LEG CGM, RIGHT LEG CGM, LEFT/RIGHT STOMACH CGM KETONES NEGATIVE, TRACE, SMALL, MODERATE, LARGE	HYDRATE 2AM BLOOD SUGAR _____ ADDITIONAL BLOOD SUGAR READINGS BS ___ at __ : __ AM/PM BS ___ at __ : __ AM/PM	NOTES MEDICINE

DATE: ______________________ SUN MON TUES WED THUR FRI SAT

	MEALS AND SNACKS	CARB AND FOOD CALCULATIONS	SHOT DETAILS AND LOCATION
BREAKFAST	Total Carbohydrates : ___._ grams	Correction Dose: (BS - ___) / __ (___-___)/__ = (__/__) = ___.__ Carb Dose Calculation: (Meal Carbs / ___) (__._ /___) = ___.__ Correction Dose + Carb Dose Calculation: (___.__ + ___.__) = __.__ OR __ UNITS Correction Dose Dose Calculation Rounded to nearest whole number	TIME __ : __ AM / PM LEFT ARM CGM / RIGHT ARM CGM / LEFT LEG CGM / RIGHT LEG CGM / LEFT/RIGHT STOMACH CGM KETONES NEGATIVE TRACE SMALL MODERATE LARGE
SNACK	Total Carbohydrates : ___._ grams	Carb Dose Calculation: (Meal Carbs / ___) (__._ /___) = ___.__ or __ UNITS NO INSULIN DOSE REQUIRED FOR MEALS/SNACKS UNDER __G OF CARBS OR EQUAL TO __.__ OR LESS	TIME __ : __ AM / PM LEFT ARM CGM / RIGHT ARM CGM / LEFT LEG CGM / RIGHT LEG CGM / LEFT/RIGHT STOMACH CGM KETONES NEGATIVE TRACE SMALL MODERATE LARGE
LUNCH	Total Carbohydrates : ___._ grams	Correction Dose: (BS - ___) / __ (___-___)/__ = (__/__) = ___.__ Carb Dose Calculation: (Meal Carbs / ___) (__._ /___) = ___.__ Correction Dose + Carb Dose Calculation: (___.__ + ___.__) = __.__ OR __ UNITS Correction Dose Dose Calculation Rounded to nearest whole number	TIME __ : __ AM / PM LEFT ARM CGM / RIGHT ARM CGM / LEFT LEG CGM / RIGHT LEG CGM / LEFT/RIGHT STOMACH CGM KETONES NEGATIVE TRACE SMALL MODERATE LARGE
SNACK	Total Carbohydrates : ___._ grams	Carb Dose Calculation: (Meal Carbs / ___) (__._ /___) = ___.__ or __ UNITS NO INSULIN DOSE REQUIRED FOR MEALS/SNACKS UNDER __G OF CARBS OR EQUAL TO __.__ OR LESS	TIME __ : __ AM / PM LEFT ARM CGM / RIGHT ARM CGM / LEFT LEG CGM / RIGHT LEG CGM / LEFT/RIGHT STOMACH CGM KETONES NEGATIVE TRACE SMALL MODERATE LARGE
DINNER	Total Carbohydrates : ___._ grams	Correction Dose: (BS - ___) / __ (___-___)/__ = (__/__) = ___.__ Carb Dose Calculation: (Meal Carbs / ___) (__._ /___) = ___.__ Correction Dose + Carb Dose Calculation: (___.__ + ___.__) = __.__ OR __ UNITS Correction Dose Dose Calculation Rounded to nearest whole number	TIME __ : __ AM / PM LEFT ARM CGM / RIGHT ARM CGM / LEFT LEG CGM / RIGHT LEG CGM / LEFT/RIGHT STOMACH CGM KETONES NEGATIVE TRACE SMALL MODERATE LARGE
SNACK	Total Carbohydrates : ___._ grams	Carb Dose Calculation: (Meal Carbs / ___) (__._ /___) = ___.__ or __ UNITS NO INSULIN DOSE REQUIRED FOR MEALS/SNACKS UNDER __G OF CARBS OR EQUAL TO __.__ OR LESS	TIME __ : __ AM / PM LEFT ARM CGM / RIGHT ARM CGM / LEFT LEG CGM / RIGHT LEG CGM / LEFT/RIGHT STOMACH CGM KETONES NEGATIVE TRACE SMALL MODERATE LARGE
BEDTIME __ : __ PM	BLOOD SUGAR _____ UNITS ___ LEFT ARM CGM / RIGHT ARM CGM / LEFT LEG CGM / RIGHT LEG CGM / LEFT/RIGHT STOMACH CGM KETONES NEGATIVE TRACE SMALL MODERATE LARGE	HYDRATE 2AM BLOOD SUGAR _____ ADDITIONAL BLOOD SUGAR READINGS BS ___ at __ : __ AM/PM BS ___ at __ : __ AM/PM	NOTES MEDICINE

DATE: ______________________________ SUN MON TUES WED THUR FRI SAT

	MEALS AND SNACKS	CARB AND FOOD CALCULATIONS	SHOT DETAILS AND LOCATION
BREAKFAST	Total Carbohydrates : ____._ grams	Correction Dose: (BS - ___) / __ (___-___)/__ = (__/__) = ___.__ Carb Dose Calculation: (Meal Carbs / ___) (__._ /___) = ___.__ Correction Dose + Carb Dose Calculation: (____.__ + ____.__) = __.__ OR __ UNITS Correction Dose · Dose Calculation · Rounded to nearest whole number	TIME __ : __ AM / PM LEFT ARM CGM · RIGHT ARM CGM · LEFT LEG CGM · RIGHT LEG CGM · LEFT/RIGHT STOMACH CGM KETONES NEGATIVE · TRACE · SMALL · MODERATE · LARGE
SNACK	Total Carbohydrates : ____._ grams	Carb Dose Calculation: (Meal Carbs / ___) (__._ /___) = ___.__ or __ UNITS NO INSULIN DOSE REQUIRED FOR MEALS/SNACKS UNDER __G OF CARBS OR EQUAL TO __.__ OR LESS	TIME __ : __ AM / PM LEFT ARM CGM · RIGHT ARM CGM · LEFT LEG CGM · RIGHT LEG CGM · LEFT/RIGHT STOMACH CGM KETONES NEGATIVE · TRACE · SMALL · MODERATE · LARGE
LUNCH	Total Carbohydrates : ____._ grams	Correction Dose: (BS - ___) / __ (___-___)/__ = (__/__) = ___.__ Carb Dose Calculation: (Meal Carbs / ___) (__._ /___) = ___.__ Correction Dose + Carb Dose Calculation: (____.__ + ____.__) = __.__ OR __ UNITS Correction Dose · Dose Calculation · Rounded to nearest whole number	TIME __ : __ AM / PM LEFT ARM CGM · RIGHT ARM CGM · LEFT LEG CGM · RIGHT LEG CGM · LEFT/RIGHT STOMACH CGM KETONES NEGATIVE · TRACE · SMALL · MODERATE · LARGE
SNACK	Total Carbohydrates : ____._ grams	Carb Dose Calculation: (Meal Carbs / ___) (__._ /___) = ___.__ or __ UNITS NO INSULIN DOSE REQUIRED FOR MEALS/SNACKS UNDER __G OF CARBS OR EQUAL TO __.__ OR LESS	TIME __ : __ AM / PM LEFT ARM CGM · RIGHT ARM CGM · LEFT LEG CGM · RIGHT LEG CGM · LEFT/RIGHT STOMACH CGM KETONES NEGATIVE · TRACE · SMALL · MODERATE · LARGE
DINNER	Total Carbohydrates : ____._ grams	Correction Dose: (BS - ___) / __ (___-___)/__ = (__/__) = ___.__ Carb Dose Calculation: (Meal Carbs / ___) (__._ /___) = ___.__ Correction Dose + Carb Dose Calculation: (____.__ + ____.__) = __.__ OR __ UNITS Correction Dose · Dose Calculation · Rounded to nearest whole number	TIME __ : __ AM / PM LEFT ARM CGM · RIGHT ARM CGM · LEFT LEG CGM · RIGHT LEG CGM · LEFT/RIGHT STOMACH CGM KETONES NEGATIVE · TRACE · SMALL · MODERATE · LARGE
SNACK	Total Carbohydrates : ____._ grams	Carb Dose Calculation: (Meal Carbs / ___) (__._ /___) = ___.__ or __ UNITS NO INSULIN DOSE REQUIRED FOR MEALS/SNACKS UNDER __G OF CARBS OR EQUAL TO __.__ OR LESS	TIME __ : __ AM / PM LEFT ARM CGM · RIGHT ARM CGM · LEFT LEG CGM · RIGHT LEG CGM · LEFT/RIGHT STOMACH CGM KETONES NEGATIVE · TRACE · SMALL · MODERATE · LARGE
BEDTIME __ : __ PM	BLOOD SUGAR _____ UNITS ___ LEFT ARM CGM · RIGHT ARM CGM · LEFT LEG CGM · RIGHT LEG CGM · LEFT/RIGHT STOMACH CGM KETONES NEGATIVE · TRACE · SMALL · MODERATE · LARGE	HYDRATE 2AM BLOOD SUGAR _____ ADDITIONAL BLOOD SUGAR READINGS BS ___ at __ : __ AM/PM BS ___ at __ : __ AM/PM	NOTES MEDICINE

DATE: ______________________ SUN MON TUES WED THUR FRI SAT

	MEALS AND SNACKS	CARB AND FOOD CALCULATIONS	SHOT DETAILS AND LOCATION
BREAKFAST	Total Carbohydrates : ___._ grams	Correction Dose: (BS - ___) / __ (___-___)/__ = (__/__) = ___.__ Carb Dose Calculation: (Meal Carbs / ___) (__._ /___) = ___.__ Correction Dose + Carb Dose Calculation: (___.__ + ___.__) = __.__ OR __ UNITS Correction Dose / Dose Calculation / Rounded to nearest whole number	TIME __ : __ AM / PM LEFT ARM CGM / RIGHT ARM CGM / LEFT LEG CGM / RIGHT LEG CGM / LEFT/RIGHT STOMACH CGM KETONES NEGATIVE / TRACE / SMALL / MODERATE / LARGE
SNACK	Total Carbohydrates : ___._ grams	Carb Dose Calculation: (Meal Carbs / ___) (__._ /___) = ___.__ or __ UNITS NO INSULIN DOSE REQUIRED FOR MEALS/SNACKS UNDER __G OF CARBS OR EQUAL TO __.__ OR LESS	TIME __ : __ AM / PM LEFT ARM CGM / RIGHT ARM CGM / LEFT LEG CGM / RIGHT LEG CGM / LEFT/RIGHT STOMACH CGM KETONES NEGATIVE / TRACE / SMALL / MODERATE / LARGE
LUNCH	Total Carbohydrates : ___._ grams	Correction Dose: (BS - ___) / __ (___-___)/__ = (__/__) = ___.__ Carb Dose Calculation: (Meal Carbs / ___) (__._ /___) = ___.__ Correction Dose + Carb Dose Calculation: (___.__ + ___.__) = __.__ OR __ UNITS Correction Dose / Dose Calculation / Rounded to nearest whole number	TIME __ : __ AM / PM LEFT ARM CGM / RIGHT ARM CGM / LEFT LEG CGM / RIGHT LEG CGM / LEFT/RIGHT STOMACH CGM KETONES NEGATIVE / TRACE / SMALL / MODERATE / LARGE
SNACK	Total Carbohydrates : ___._ grams	Carb Dose Calculation: (Meal Carbs / ___) (__._ /___) = ___.__ or __ UNITS NO INSULIN DOSE REQUIRED FOR MEALS/SNACKS UNDER __G OF CARBS OR EQUAL TO __.__ OR LESS	TIME __ : __ AM / PM LEFT ARM CGM / RIGHT ARM CGM / LEFT LEG CGM / RIGHT LEG CGM / LEFT/RIGHT STOMACH CGM KETONES NEGATIVE / TRACE / SMALL / MODERATE / LARGE
DINNER	Total Carbohydrates : ___._ grams	Correction Dose: (BS - ___) / __ (___-___)/__ = (__/__) = ___.__ Carb Dose Calculation: (Meal Carbs / ___) (__._ /___) = ___.__ Correction Dose + Carb Dose Calculation: (___.__ + ___.__) = __.__ OR __ UNITS Correction Dose / Dose Calculation / Rounded to nearest whole number	TIME __ : __ AM / PM LEFT ARM CGM / RIGHT ARM CGM / LEFT LEG CGM / RIGHT LEG CGM / LEFT/RIGHT STOMACH CGM KETONES NEGATIVE / TRACE / SMALL / MODERATE / LARGE
SNACK	Total Carbohydrates : ___._ grams	Carb Dose Calculation: (Meal Carbs / ___) (__._ /___) = ___.__ or __ UNITS NO INSULIN DOSE REQUIRED FOR MEALS/SNACKS UNDER __G OF CARBS OR EQUAL TO __.__ OR LESS	TIME __ : __ AM / PM LEFT ARM CGM / RIGHT ARM CGM / LEFT LEG CGM / RIGHT LEG CGM / LEFT/RIGHT STOMACH CGM KETONES NEGATIVE / TRACE / SMALL / MODERATE / LARGE
BEDTIME __ : __ PM	BLOOD SUGAR ____ UNITS ___ LEFT ARM CGM / RIGHT ARM CGM / LEFT LEG CGM / RIGHT LEG CGM / LEFT/RIGHT STOMACH CGM KETONES NEGATIVE / TRACE / SMALL / MODERATE / LARGE	HYDRATE 2AM BLOOD SUGAR ____ ADDITIONAL BLOOD SUGAR READINGS BS ___ at __ : __ AM/PM BS ___ at __ : __ AM/PM	NOTES MEDICINE

DATE: ______________________ SUN MON TUES WED THUR FRI SAT

	MEALS AND SNACKS	CARB AND FOOD CALCULATIONS	SHOT DETAILS AND LOCATION
BREAKFAST	Total Carbohydrates : ___.__ grams	Correction Dose: (BS - ___) / __ (___-___)/__ = (__/__) = ___.__ Carb Dose Calculation: (Meal Carbs / ___) (__.__ /___) = ___.__ Correction Dose + Carb Dose Calculation: (______ + ______) = __.__ OR __ UNITS Correction Dose / Dose Calculation / Rounded to nearest whole number	TIME __ : __ AM / PM LEFT ARM CGM / RIGHT ARM CGM / LEFT LEG CGM / RIGHT LEG CGM / LEFT/RIGHT STOMACH CGM KETONES NEGATIVE TRACE SMALL MODERATE LARGE
SNACK	Total Carbohydrates : ___.__ grams	Carb Dose Calculation: (Meal Carbs / ___) (__.__ /___) = ___.__ or __ UNITS NO INSULIN DOSE REQUIRED FOR MEALS/SNACKS UNDER __G OF CARBS OR EQUAL TO __.__ OR LESS	TIME __ : __ AM / PM LEFT ARM CGM / RIGHT ARM CGM / LEFT LEG CGM / RIGHT LEG CGM / LEFT/RIGHT STOMACH CGM KETONES NEGATIVE TRACE SMALL MODERATE LARGE
LUNCH	Total Carbohydrates : ___.__ grams	Correction Dose: (BS - ___) / __ (___-___)/__ = (__/__) = ___.__ Carb Dose Calculation: (Meal Carbs / ___) (__.__ /___) = ___.__ Correction Dose + Carb Dose Calculation: (______ + ______) = __.__ OR __ UNITS Correction Dose / Dose Calculation / Rounded to nearest whole number	TIME __ : __ AM / PM LEFT ARM CGM / RIGHT ARM CGM / LEFT LEG CGM / RIGHT LEG CGM / LEFT/RIGHT STOMACH CGM KETONES NEGATIVE TRACE SMALL MODERATE LARGE
SNACK	Total Carbohydrates : ___.__ grams	Carb Dose Calculation: (Meal Carbs / ___) (__.__ /___) = ___.__ or __ UNITS NO INSULIN DOSE REQUIRED FOR MEALS/SNACKS UNDER __G OF CARBS OR EQUAL TO __.__ OR LESS	TIME __ : __ AM / PM LEFT ARM CGM / RIGHT ARM CGM / LEFT LEG CGM / RIGHT LEG CGM / LEFT/RIGHT STOMACH CGM KETONES NEGATIVE TRACE SMALL MODERATE LARGE
DINNER	Total Carbohydrates : ___.__ grams	Correction Dose: (BS - ___) / __ (___-___)/__ = (__/__) = ___.__ Carb Dose Calculation: (Meal Carbs / ___) (__.__ /___) = ___.__ Correction Dose + Carb Dose Calculation: (______ + ______) = __.__ OR __ UNITS Correction Dose / Dose Calculation / Rounded to nearest whole number	TIME __ : __ AM / PM LEFT ARM CGM / RIGHT ARM CGM / LEFT LEG CGM / RIGHT LEG CGM / LEFT/RIGHT STOMACH CGM KETONES NEGATIVE TRACE SMALL MODERATE LARGE
SNACK	Total Carbohydrates : ___.__ grams	Carb Dose Calculation: (Meal Carbs / ___) (__.__ /___) = ___.__ or __ UNITS NO INSULIN DOSE REQUIRED FOR MEALS/SNACKS UNDER __G OF CARBS OR EQUAL TO __.__ OR LESS	TIME __ : __ AM / PM LEFT ARM CGM / RIGHT ARM CGM / LEFT LEG CGM / RIGHT LEG CGM / LEFT/RIGHT STOMACH CGM KETONES NEGATIVE TRACE SMALL MODERATE LARGE
BEDTIME __ : __ PM	BLOOD SUGAR ____ UNITS ___ LEFT ARM CGM / RIGHT ARM CGM / LEFT LEG CGM / RIGHT LEG CGM / LEFT/RIGHT STOMACH CGM KETONES NEGATIVE TRACE SMALL MODERATE LARGE	HYDRATE 2AM BLOOD SUGAR ____ ADDITIONAL BLOOD SUGAR READINGS BS ___ at __ : __ AM/PM BS ___ at __ : __ AM/PM	NOTES MEDICINE

DATE: ______________________________ SUN MON TUES WED THUR FRI SAT

	MEALS AND SNACKS	CARB AND FOOD CALCULATIONS	SHOT DETAILS AND LOCATION
BREAKFAST	Total Carbohydrates : ___._ grams	Correction Dose: (BS - ___) / __ (___-___)/__ = (__/__) = ___.__ Carb Dose Calculation: (Meal Carbs / ___) (__._ /___) = ___.__ Correction Dose + Carb Dose Calculation: (__.__ + __.__) = __.__ OR __ UNITS Correction Dose / Dose Calculation / Rounded to nearest whole number	TIME __ : __ AM / PM LEFT ARM CGM / RIGHT ARM CGM / LEFT LEG CGM / RIGHT LEG CGM / LEFT/RIGHT STOMACH CGM KETONES NEGATIVE / TRACE / SMALL / MODERATE / LARGE
SNACK	Total Carbohydrates : ___._ grams	Carb Dose Calculation: (Meal Carbs / ___) (__._ /___) = ___.__ or __ UNITS NO INSULIN DOSE REQUIRED FOR MEALS/SNACKS UNDER __G OF CARBS OR EQUAL TO __.__ OR LESS	TIME __ : __ AM / PM LEFT ARM CGM / RIGHT ARM CGM / LEFT LEG CGM / RIGHT LEG CGM / LEFT/RIGHT STOMACH CGM KETONES NEGATIVE / TRACE / SMALL / MODERATE / LARGE
LUNCH	Total Carbohydrates : ___._ grams	Correction Dose: (BS - ___) / __ (___-___)/__ = (__/__) = ___.__ Carb Dose Calculation: (Meal Carbs / ___) (__._ /___) = ___.__ Correction Dose + Carb Dose Calculation: (__.__ + __.__) = __.__ OR __ UNITS Correction Dose / Dose Calculation / Rounded to nearest whole number	TIME __ : __ AM / PM LEFT ARM CGM / RIGHT ARM CGM / LEFT LEG CGM / RIGHT LEG CGM / LEFT/RIGHT STOMACH CGM KETONES NEGATIVE / TRACE / SMALL / MODERATE / LARGE
SNACK	Total Carbohydrates : ___._ grams	Carb Dose Calculation: (Meal Carbs / ___) (__._ /___) = ___.__ or __ UNITS NO INSULIN DOSE REQUIRED FOR MEALS/SNACKS UNDER __G OF CARBS OR EQUAL TO __.__ OR LESS	TIME __ : __ AM / PM LEFT ARM CGM / RIGHT ARM CGM / LEFT LEG CGM / RIGHT LEG CGM / LEFT/RIGHT STOMACH CGM KETONES NEGATIVE / TRACE / SMALL / MODERATE / LARGE
DINNER	Total Carbohydrates : ___._ grams	Correction Dose: (BS - ___) / __ (___-___)/__ = (__/__) = ___.__ Carb Dose Calculation: (Meal Carbs / ___) (__._ /___) = ___.__ Correction Dose + Carb Dose Calculation: (__.__ + __.__) = __.__ OR __ UNITS Correction Dose / Dose Calculation / Rounded to nearest whole number	TIME __ : __ AM / PM LEFT ARM CGM / RIGHT ARM CGM / LEFT LEG CGM / RIGHT LEG CGM / LEFT/RIGHT STOMACH CGM KETONES NEGATIVE / TRACE / SMALL / MODERATE / LARGE
SNACK	Total Carbohydrates : ___._ grams	Carb Dose Calculation: (Meal Carbs / ___) (__._ /___) = ___.__ or __ UNITS NO INSULIN DOSE REQUIRED FOR MEALS/SNACKS UNDER __G OF CARBS OR EQUAL TO __.__ OR LESS	TIME __ : __ AM / PM LEFT ARM CGM / RIGHT ARM CGM / LEFT LEG CGM / RIGHT LEG CGM / LEFT/RIGHT STOMACH CGM KETONES NEGATIVE / TRACE / SMALL / MODERATE / LARGE
BEDTIME __ : __ PM	BLOOD SUGAR _____ UNITS ___ LEFT ARM CGM / RIGHT ARM CGM / LEFT LEG CGM / RIGHT LEG CGM / LEFT/RIGHT STOMACH CGM KETONES NEGATIVE / TRACE / SMALL / MODERATE / LARGE	HYDRATE 2AM BLOOD SUGAR _____ ADDITIONAL BLOOD SUGAR READINGS BS ___ at __ : __ AM/PM BS ___ at __ : __ AM/PM	NOTES MEDICINE

DATE: ____________________ SUN MON TUES WED THUR FRI SAT

	MEALS AND SNACKS	CARB AND FOOD CALCULATIONS	SHOT DETAILS AND LOCATION
BREAKFAST	Total Carbohydrates : ___._ grams	Correction Dose: (BS - ___) / __ (___-___)/__ = (__/__) = ___.__ Carb Dose Calculation: (Meal Carbs / ___) (__._ /___) = ___.__ Correction Dose + Carb Dose Calculation: (_____ + _____) = ___.__ OR __ UNITS Correction Dose / Dose Calculation / Rounded to nearest whole number	TIME __ : __ AM / PM LEFT ARM CGM / RIGHT ARM CGM / LEFT LEG CGM / RIGHT LEG CGM / LEFT/RIGHT STOMACH CGM KETONES NEGATIVE / TRACE / SMALL / MODERATE / LARGE
SNACK	Total Carbohydrates : ___._ grams	Carb Dose Calculation: (Meal Carbs / ___) (__._ /___) = ___.__ or __ UNITS NO INSULIN DOSE REQUIRED FOR MEALS/SNACKS UNDER __G OF CARBS OR EQUAL TO __.__ OR LESS	TIME __ : __ AM / PM LEFT ARM CGM / RIGHT ARM CGM / LEFT LEG CGM / RIGHT LEG CGM / LEFT/RIGHT STOMACH CGM KETONES NEGATIVE / TRACE / SMALL / MODERATE / LARGE
LUNCH	Total Carbohydrates : ___._ grams	Correction Dose: (BS - ___) / __ (___-___)/__ = (__/__) = ___.__ Carb Dose Calculation: (Meal Carbs / ___) (__._ /___) = ___.__ Correction Dose + Carb Dose Calculation: (_____ + _____) = ___.__ OR __ UNITS Correction Dose / Dose Calculation / Rounded to nearest whole number	TIME __ : __ AM / PM LEFT ARM CGM / RIGHT ARM CGM / LEFT LEG CGM / RIGHT LEG CGM / LEFT/RIGHT STOMACH CGM KETONES NEGATIVE / TRACE / SMALL / MODERATE / LARGE
SNACK	Total Carbohydrates : ___._ grams	Carb Dose Calculation: (Meal Carbs / ___) (__._ /___) = ___.__ or __ UNITS NO INSULIN DOSE REQUIRED FOR MEALS/SNACKS UNDER __G OF CARBS OR EQUAL TO __.__ OR LESS	TIME __ : __ AM / PM LEFT ARM CGM / RIGHT ARM CGM / LEFT LEG CGM / RIGHT LEG CGM / LEFT/RIGHT STOMACH CGM KETONES NEGATIVE / TRACE / SMALL / MODERATE / LARGE
DINNER	Total Carbohydrates : ___._ grams	Correction Dose: (BS - ___) / __ (___-___)/__ = (__/__) = ___.__ Carb Dose Calculation: (Meal Carbs / ___) (__._ /___) = ___.__ Correction Dose + Carb Dose Calculation: (_____ + _____) = ___.__ OR __ UNITS Correction Dose / Dose Calculation / Rounded to nearest whole number	TIME __ : __ AM / PM LEFT ARM CGM / RIGHT ARM CGM / LEFT LEG CGM / RIGHT LEG CGM / LEFT/RIGHT STOMACH CGM KETONES NEGATIVE / TRACE / SMALL / MODERATE / LARGE
SNACK	Total Carbohydrates : ___._ grams	Carb Dose Calculation: (Meal Carbs / ___) (__._ /___) = ___.__ or __ UNITS NO INSULIN DOSE REQUIRED FOR MEALS/SNACKS UNDER __G OF CARBS OR EQUAL TO __.__ OR LESS	TIME __ : __ AM / PM LEFT ARM CGM / RIGHT ARM CGM / LEFT LEG CGM / RIGHT LEG CGM / LEFT/RIGHT STOMACH CGM KETONES NEGATIVE / TRACE / SMALL / MODERATE / LARGE
BEDTIME __ : __ PM	BLOOD SUGAR ______ UNITS ___ LEFT ARM CGM / RIGHT ARM CGM / LEFT LEG CGM / RIGHT LEG CGM / LEFT/RIGHT STOMACH CGM KETONES NEGATIVE / TRACE / SMALL / MODERATE / LARGE	HYDRATE 2AM BLOOD SUGAR _____ ADDITIONAL BLOOD SUGAR READINGS BS ___ at __ : __ AM/PM BS ___ at __ : __ AM/PM	NOTES MEDICINE

DATE: ______________________________ SUN MON TUES WED THUR FRI SAT

	MEALS AND SNACKS	CARB AND FOOD CALCULATIONS	SHOT DETAILS AND LOCATION
BREAKFAST	Total Carbohydrates : ___._ grams	Correction Dose: (BS - ___) / __ (___-___)/__ = (__/__) = ___.__ Carb Dose Calculation: (Meal Carbs / ___) (__._ /___) = ___.__ Correction Dose + Carb Dose Calculation: (___.__ + ___.__) = __.__ OR __ UNITS Correction Dose · Dose Calculation · Rounded to nearest whole number	TIME __ : __ AM / PM LEFT ARM CGM · RIGHT ARM CGM · LEFT LEG CGM · RIGHT LEG CGM · LEFT/RIGHT STOMACH CGM KETONES NEGATIVE · TRACE · SMALL · MODERATE · LARGE
SNACK	Total Carbohydrates : ___._ grams	Carb Dose Calculation: (Meal Carbs / ___) (__._ /___) = ___.__ or __ UNITS NO INSULIN DOSE REQUIRED FOR MEALS/SNACKS UNDER __G OF CARBS OR EQUAL TO __.__ OR LESS	TIME __ : __ AM / PM LEFT ARM CGM · RIGHT ARM CGM · LEFT LEG CGM · RIGHT LEG CGM · LEFT/RIGHT STOMACH CGM KETONES NEGATIVE · TRACE · SMALL · MODERATE · LARGE
LUNCH	Total Carbohydrates : ___._ grams	Correction Dose: (BS - ___) / __ (___-___)/__ = (__/__) = ___.__ Carb Dose Calculation: (Meal Carbs / ___) (__._ /___) = ___.__ Correction Dose + Carb Dose Calculation: (___.__ + ___.__) = __.__ OR __ UNITS Correction Dose · Dose Calculation · Rounded to nearest whole number	TIME __ : __ AM / PM LEFT ARM CGM · RIGHT ARM CGM · LEFT LEG CGM · RIGHT LEG CGM · LEFT/RIGHT STOMACH CGM KETONES NEGATIVE · TRACE · SMALL · MODERATE · LARGE
SNACK	Total Carbohydrates : ___._ grams	Carb Dose Calculation: (Meal Carbs / ___) (__._ /___) = ___.__ or __ UNITS NO INSULIN DOSE REQUIRED FOR MEALS/SNACKS UNDER __G OF CARBS OR EQUAL TO __.__ OR LESS	TIME __ : __ AM / PM LEFT ARM CGM · RIGHT ARM CGM · LEFT LEG CGM · RIGHT LEG CGM · LEFT/RIGHT STOMACH CGM KETONES NEGATIVE · TRACE · SMALL · MODERATE · LARGE
DINNER	Total Carbohydrates : ___._ grams	Correction Dose: (BS - ___) / __ (___-___)/__ = (__/__) = ___.__ Carb Dose Calculation: (Meal Carbs / ___) (__._ /___) = ___.__ Correction Dose + Carb Dose Calculation: (___.__ + ___.__) = __.__ OR __ UNITS Correction Dose · Dose Calculation · Rounded to nearest whole number	TIME __ : __ AM / PM LEFT ARM CGM · RIGHT ARM CGM · LEFT LEG CGM · RIGHT LEG CGM · LEFT/RIGHT STOMACH CGM KETONES NEGATIVE · TRACE · SMALL · MODERATE · LARGE
SNACK	Total Carbohydrates : ___._ grams	Carb Dose Calculation: (Meal Carbs / ___) (__._ /___) = ___.__ or __ UNITS NO INSULIN DOSE REQUIRED FOR MEALS/SNACKS UNDER __G OF CARBS OR EQUAL TO __.__ OR LESS	TIME __ : __ AM / PM LEFT ARM CGM · RIGHT ARM CGM · LEFT LEG CGM · RIGHT LEG CGM · LEFT/RIGHT STOMACH CGM KETONES NEGATIVE · TRACE · SMALL · MODERATE · LARGE
BEDTIME __ : __ PM	BLOOD SUGAR ____ UNITS ___ LEFT ARM CGM · RIGHT ARM CGM · LEFT LEG CGM · RIGHT LEG CGM · LEFT/RIGHT STOMACH CGM KETONES NEGATIVE · TRACE · SMALL · MODERATE · LARGE	HYDRATE 2AM BLOOD SUGAR ____ ADDITIONAL BLOOD SUGAR READINGS BS ___ at __ : __ AM/PM BS ___ at __ : __ AM/PM	NOTES MEDICINE

DATE: ______________________ SUN MON TUES WED THUR FRI SAT

	MEALS AND SNACKS	CARB AND FOOD CALCULATIONS	SHOT DETAILS AND LOCATION
BREAKFAST	Total Carbohydrates : ____._ grams	Correction Dose: (BS - ___) / __ (___-___)/__ = (__/__) = ____.__ Carb Dose Calculation: (Meal Carbs / ___) (__._ /___) = ____.__ Correction Dose + Carb Dose Calculation: (_____ + _____) = __.__ OR __ UNITS Correction Dose / Dose Calculation / Rounded to nearest whole number	TIME __ : __ AM / PM LEFT ARM CGM / RIGHT ARM CGM / LEFT LEG CGM / RIGHT LEG CGM / LEFT/RIGHT STOMACH CGM KETONES NEGATIVE / TRACE / SMALL / MODERATE / LARGE
SNACK	Total Carbohydrates : ____._ grams	Carb Dose Calculation: (Meal Carbs / ___) (__._ /___) = ____.__ or __ UNITS NO INSULIN DOSE REQUIRED FOR MEALS/SNACKS UNDER __G OF CARBS OR EQUAL TO __.__ OR LESS	TIME __ : __ AM / PM LEFT ARM CGM / RIGHT ARM CGM / LEFT LEG CGM / RIGHT LEG CGM / LEFT/RIGHT STOMACH CGM KETONES NEGATIVE / TRACE / SMALL / MODERATE / LARGE
LUNCH	Total Carbohydrates : ____._ grams	Correction Dose: (BS - ___) / __ (___-___)/__ = (__/__) = ____.__ Carb Dose Calculation: (Meal Carbs / ___) (__._ /___) = ____.__ Correction Dose + Carb Dose Calculation: (_____ + _____) = __.__ OR __ UNITS Correction Dose / Dose Calculation / Rounded to nearest whole number	TIME __ : __ AM / PM LEFT ARM CGM / RIGHT ARM CGM / LEFT LEG CGM / RIGHT LEG CGM / LEFT/RIGHT STOMACH CGM KETONES NEGATIVE / TRACE / SMALL / MODERATE / LARGE
SNACK	Total Carbohydrates : ____._ grams	Carb Dose Calculation: (Meal Carbs / ___) (__._ /___) = ____.__ or __ UNITS NO INSULIN DOSE REQUIRED FOR MEALS/SNACKS UNDER __G OF CARBS OR EQUAL TO __.__ OR LESS	TIME __ : __ AM / PM LEFT ARM CGM / RIGHT ARM CGM / LEFT LEG CGM / RIGHT LEG CGM / LEFT/RIGHT STOMACH CGM KETONES NEGATIVE / TRACE / SMALL / MODERATE / LARGE
DINNER	Total Carbohydrates : ____._ grams	Correction Dose: (BS - ___) / __ (___-___)/__ = (__/__) = ____.__ Carb Dose Calculation: (Meal Carbs / ___) (__._ /___) = ____.__ Correction Dose + Carb Dose Calculation: (_____ + _____) = __.__ OR __ UNITS Correction Dose / Dose Calculation / Rounded to nearest whole number	TIME __ : __ AM / PM LEFT ARM CGM / RIGHT ARM CGM / LEFT LEG CGM / RIGHT LEG CGM / LEFT/RIGHT STOMACH CGM KETONES NEGATIVE / TRACE / SMALL / MODERATE / LARGE
SNACK	Total Carbohydrates : ____._ grams	Carb Dose Calculation: (Meal Carbs / ___) (__._ /___) = ____.__ or __ UNITS NO INSULIN DOSE REQUIRED FOR MEALS/SNACKS UNDER __G OF CARBS OR EQUAL TO __.__ OR LESS	TIME __ : __ AM / PM LEFT ARM CGM / RIGHT ARM CGM / LEFT LEG CGM / RIGHT LEG CGM / LEFT/RIGHT STOMACH CGM KETONES NEGATIVE / TRACE / SMALL / MODERATE / LARGE
BEDTIME __ : __ PM	BLOOD SUGAR ____ UNITS ___ LEFT ARM CGM / RIGHT ARM CGM / LEFT LEG CGM / RIGHT LEG CGM / LEFT/RIGHT STOMACH CGM KETONES NEGATIVE / TRACE / SMALL / MODERATE / LARGE	HYDRATE 2AM BLOOD SUGAR ____ ADDITIONAL BLOOD SUGAR READINGS BS ___ at __ : __ AM/PM BS ___ at __ : __ AM/PM	NOTES MEDICINE

DATE: ______________________________ SUN MON TUES WED THUR FRI SAT

	MEALS AND SNACKS	CARB AND FOOD CALCULATIONS	SHOT DETAILS AND LOCATION
BREAKFAST	Total Carbohydrates : ___._ grams	Correction Dose: (BS - ___) / __ (___-___)/__ = (__/__) = ___.__ Carb Dose Calculation: (Meal Carbs / ___) (__._ /___) = ___.__ Correction Dose + Carb Dose Calculation: (___.__ + ___.__) = __.__ OR __ UNITS Correction Dose / Dose Calculation / Rounded to nearest whole number	TIME __ : __ AM / PM LEFT ARM CGM / RIGHT ARM CGM / LEFT LEG CGM / RIGHT LEG CGM / LEFT/RIGHT STOMACH CGM KETONES NEGATIVE / TRACE / SMALL / MODERATE / LARGE
SNACK	Total Carbohydrates : ___._ grams	Carb Dose Calculation: (Meal Carbs / ___) (__._ /___) = ___.__ or __ UNITS NO INSULIN DOSE REQUIRED FOR MEALS/SNACKS UNDER __G OF CARBS OR EQUAL TO __.__ OR LESS	TIME __ : __ AM / PM LEFT ARM CGM / RIGHT ARM CGM / LEFT LEG CGM / RIGHT LEG CGM / LEFT/RIGHT STOMACH CGM KETONES NEGATIVE / TRACE / SMALL / MODERATE / LARGE
LUNCH	Total Carbohydrates : ___._ grams	Correction Dose: (BS - ___) / __ (___-___)/__ = (__/__) = ___.__ Carb Dose Calculation: (Meal Carbs / ___) (__._ /___) = ___.__ Correction Dose + Carb Dose Calculation: (___.__ + ___.__) = __.__ OR __ UNITS Correction Dose / Dose Calculation / Rounded to nearest whole number	TIME __ : __ AM / PM LEFT ARM CGM / RIGHT ARM CGM / LEFT LEG CGM / RIGHT LEG CGM / LEFT/RIGHT STOMACH CGM KETONES NEGATIVE / TRACE / SMALL / MODERATE / LARGE
SNACK	Total Carbohydrates : ___._ grams	Carb Dose Calculation: (Meal Carbs / ___) (__._ /___) = ___.__ or __ UNITS NO INSULIN DOSE REQUIRED FOR MEALS/SNACKS UNDER __G OF CARBS OR EQUAL TO __.__ OR LESS	TIME __ : __ AM / PM LEFT ARM CGM / RIGHT ARM CGM / LEFT LEG CGM / RIGHT LEG CGM / LEFT/RIGHT STOMACH CGM KETONES NEGATIVE / TRACE / SMALL / MODERATE / LARGE
DINNER	Total Carbohydrates : ___._ grams	Correction Dose: (BS - ___) / __ (___-___)/__ = (__/__) = ___.__ Carb Dose Calculation: (Meal Carbs / ___) (__._ /___) = ___.__ Correction Dose + Carb Dose Calculation: (___.__ + ___.__) = __.__ OR __ UNITS Correction Dose / Dose Calculation / Rounded to nearest whole number	TIME __ : __ AM / PM LEFT ARM CGM / RIGHT ARM CGM / LEFT LEG CGM / RIGHT LEG CGM / LEFT/RIGHT STOMACH CGM KETONES NEGATIVE / TRACE / SMALL / MODERATE / LARGE
SNACK	Total Carbohydrates : ___._ grams	Carb Dose Calculation: (Meal Carbs / ___) (__._ /___) = ___.__ or __ UNITS NO INSULIN DOSE REQUIRED FOR MEALS/SNACKS UNDER __G OF CARBS OR EQUAL TO __.__ OR LESS	TIME __ : __ AM / PM LEFT ARM CGM / RIGHT ARM CGM / LEFT LEG CGM / RIGHT LEG CGM / LEFT/RIGHT STOMACH CGM KETONES NEGATIVE / TRACE / SMALL / MODERATE / LARGE
BEDTIME __ : __ PM	BLOOD SUGAR _____ UNITS ___ LEFT ARM CGM / RIGHT ARM CGM / LEFT LEG CGM / RIGHT LEG CGM / LEFT/RIGHT STOMACH CGM KETONES NEGATIVE / TRACE / SMALL / MODERATE / LARGE	HYDRATE 2AM BLOOD SUGAR _____ ADDITIONAL BLOOD SUGAR READINGS BS ___ at __ : __ AM/PM BS ___ at __ : __ AM/PM	NOTES MEDICINE

DATE: ______________________ SUN MON TUES WED THUR FRI SAT

	MEALS AND SNACKS	CARB AND FOOD CALCULATIONS	SHOT DETAILS AND LOCATION
BREAKFAST	Total Carbohydrates : ___._ grams	Correction Dose: (BS - ___) / __ (___-___)/__ = (__/__) = ___.__ Carb Dose Calculation: (Meal Carbs / ___) (__._ /___) = ___.__ Correction Dose + Carb Dose Calculation: (___.__ + ___.__) = __.__ OR __ UNITS Correction Dose / Dose Calculation / Rounded to nearest whole number	TIME __ : __ AM / PM LEFT ARM CGM / RIGHT ARM CGM / LEFT LEG CGM / RIGHT LEG CGM / LEFT/RIGHT STOMACH CGM KETONES NEGATIVE / TRACE / SMALL / MODERATE / LARGE
SNACK	Total Carbohydrates : ___._ grams	Carb Dose Calculation: (Meal Carbs / ___) (__._ /___) = ___.__ or __ UNITS NO INSULIN DOSE REQUIRED FOR MEALS/SNACKS UNDER __G OF CARBS OR EQUAL TO __.__ OR LESS	TIME __ : __ AM / PM LEFT ARM CGM / RIGHT ARM CGM / LEFT LEG CGM / RIGHT LEG CGM / LEFT/RIGHT STOMACH CGM KETONES NEGATIVE / TRACE / SMALL / MODERATE / LARGE
LUNCH	Total Carbohydrates : ___._ grams	Correction Dose: (BS - ___) / __ (___-___)/__ = (__/__) = ___.__ Carb Dose Calculation: (Meal Carbs / ___) (__._ /___) = ___.__ Correction Dose + Carb Dose Calculation: (___.__ + ___.__) = __.__ OR __ UNITS Correction Dose / Dose Calculation / Rounded to nearest whole number	TIME __ : __ AM / PM LEFT ARM CGM / RIGHT ARM CGM / LEFT LEG CGM / RIGHT LEG CGM / LEFT/RIGHT STOMACH CGM KETONES NEGATIVE / TRACE / SMALL / MODERATE / LARGE
SNACK	Total Carbohydrates : ___._ grams	Carb Dose Calculation: (Meal Carbs / ___) (__._ /___) = ___.__ or __ UNITS NO INSULIN DOSE REQUIRED FOR MEALS/SNACKS UNDER __G OF CARBS OR EQUAL TO __.__ OR LESS	TIME __ : __ AM / PM LEFT ARM CGM / RIGHT ARM CGM / LEFT LEG CGM / RIGHT LEG CGM / LEFT/RIGHT STOMACH CGM KETONES NEGATIVE / TRACE / SMALL / MODERATE / LARGE
DINNER	Total Carbohydrates : ___._ grams	Correction Dose: (BS - ___) / __ (___-___)/__ = (__/__) = ___.__ Carb Dose Calculation: (Meal Carbs / ___) (__._ /___) = ___.__ Correction Dose + Carb Dose Calculation: (___.__ + ___.__) = __.__ OR __ UNITS Correction Dose / Dose Calculation / Rounded to nearest whole number	TIME __ : __ AM / PM LEFT ARM CGM / RIGHT ARM CGM / LEFT LEG CGM / RIGHT LEG CGM / LEFT/RIGHT STOMACH CGM KETONES NEGATIVE / TRACE / SMALL / MODERATE / LARGE
SNACK	Total Carbohydrates : ___._ grams	Carb Dose Calculation: (Meal Carbs / ___) (__._ /___) = ___.__ or __ UNITS NO INSULIN DOSE REQUIRED FOR MEALS/SNACKS UNDER __G OF CARBS OR EQUAL TO __.__ OR LESS	TIME __ : __ AM / PM LEFT ARM CGM / RIGHT ARM CGM / LEFT LEG CGM / RIGHT LEG CGM / LEFT/RIGHT STOMACH CGM KETONES NEGATIVE / TRACE / SMALL / MODERATE / LARGE
BEDTIME __ : __ PM	BLOOD SUGAR ______ UNITS ___ LEFT ARM CGM / RIGHT ARM CGM / LEFT LEG CGM / RIGHT LEG CGM / LEFT/RIGHT STOMACH CGM KETONES NEGATIVE / TRACE / SMALL / MODERATE / LARGE	HYDRATE 2AM BLOOD SUGAR _____ ADDITIONAL BLOOD SUGAR READINGS BS ___ at __ : __ AM/PM BS ___ at __ : __ AM/PM	NOTES MEDICINE

DATE: ____________________ SUN MON TUES WED THUR FRI SAT

	MEALS AND SNACKS	CARB AND FOOD CALCULATIONS	SHOT DETAILS AND LOCATION
BREAKFAST	Total Carbohydrates : ___._ grams	Correction Dose: (BS - ___) / __ (___-___)/__ = (__/__) = ___.__ Carb Dose Calculation: (Meal Carbs / ___) (__._ /___) = ___.__ Correction Dose + Carb Dose Calculation: (_____ + _____) = __.__ OR __ UNITS Correction Dose / Dose Calculation / Rounded to nearest whole number	TIME __ : __ AM / PM LEFT ARM CGM / RIGHT ARM CGM / LEFT LEG CGM / RIGHT LEG CGM / LEFT/RIGHT STOMACH CGM KETONES NEGATIVE TRACE SMALL MODERATE LARGE
SNACK	Total Carbohydrates : ___._ grams	Carb Dose Calculation: (Meal Carbs / ___) (__._ /___) = ___.__ or __ UNITS NO INSULIN DOSE REQUIRED FOR MEALS/SNACKS UNDER __G OF CARBS OR EQUAL TO __.__ OR LESS	TIME __ : __ AM / PM LEFT ARM CGM / RIGHT ARM CGM / LEFT LEG CGM / RIGHT LEG CGM / LEFT/RIGHT STOMACH CGM KETONES NEGATIVE TRACE SMALL MODERATE LARGE
LUNCH	Total Carbohydrates : ___._ grams	Correction Dose: (BS - ___) / __ (___-___)/__ = (__/__) = ___.__ Carb Dose Calculation: (Meal Carbs / ___) (__._ /___) = ___.__ Correction Dose + Carb Dose Calculation: (_____ + _____) = __.__ OR __ UNITS Correction Dose / Dose Calculation / Rounded to nearest whole number	TIME __ : __ AM / PM LEFT ARM CGM / RIGHT ARM CGM / LEFT LEG CGM / RIGHT LEG CGM / LEFT/RIGHT STOMACH CGM KETONES NEGATIVE TRACE SMALL MODERATE LARGE
SNACK	Total Carbohydrates : ___._ grams	Carb Dose Calculation: (Meal Carbs / ___) (__._ /___) = ___.__ or __ UNITS NO INSULIN DOSE REQUIRED FOR MEALS/SNACKS UNDER __G OF CARBS OR EQUAL TO __.__ OR LESS	TIME __ : __ AM / PM LEFT ARM CGM / RIGHT ARM CGM / LEFT LEG CGM / RIGHT LEG CGM / LEFT/RIGHT STOMACH CGM KETONES NEGATIVE TRACE SMALL MODERATE LARGE
DINNER	Total Carbohydrates : ___._ grams	Correction Dose: (BS - ___) / __ (___-___)/__ = (__/__) = ___.__ Carb Dose Calculation: (Meal Carbs / ___) (__._ /___) = ___.__ Correction Dose + Carb Dose Calculation: (_____ + _____) = __.__ OR __ UNITS Correction Dose / Dose Calculation / Rounded to nearest whole number	TIME __ : __ AM / PM LEFT ARM CGM / RIGHT ARM CGM / LEFT LEG CGM / RIGHT LEG CGM / LEFT/RIGHT STOMACH CGM KETONES NEGATIVE TRACE SMALL MODERATE LARGE
SNACK	Total Carbohydrates : ___._ grams	Carb Dose Calculation: (Meal Carbs / ___) (__._ /___) = ___.__ or __ UNITS NO INSULIN DOSE REQUIRED FOR MEALS/SNACKS UNDER __G OF CARBS OR EQUAL TO __.__ OR LESS	TIME __ : __ AM / PM LEFT ARM CGM / RIGHT ARM CGM / LEFT LEG CGM / RIGHT LEG CGM / LEFT/RIGHT STOMACH CGM KETONES NEGATIVE TRACE SMALL MODERATE LARGE
BEDTIME __ : __ PM	BLOOD SUGAR ____ UNITS __ LEFT ARM CGM / RIGHT ARM CGM / LEFT LEG CGM / RIGHT LEG CGM / LEFT/RIGHT STOMACH CGM KETONES NEGATIVE TRACE SMALL MODERATE LARGE	HYDRATE 2AM BLOOD SUGAR ____ ADDITIONAL BLOOD SUGAR READINGS BS ___ at __ : __ AM/PM BS ___ at __ : __ AM/PM	NOTES MEDICINE

DATE: ______________________ SUN MON TUES WED THUR FRI SAT

	MEALS AND SNACKS	CARB AND FOOD CALCULATIONS	SHOT DETAILS AND LOCATION
BREAKFAST	Total Carbohydrates : ___._ grams	Correction Dose: (BS - ___) / __ (___-___)/__ = (__/__) = ___.__ Carb Dose Calculation: (Meal Carbs / ___) (__._ /___) = ___.__ Correction Dose + Carb Dose Calculation: (___.__ + ___.__) = __.__ OR __ UNITS Correction Dose / Dose Calculation / Rounded to nearest whole number	TIME __ : __ AM / PM LEFT ARM CGM / RIGHT ARM CGM / LEFT LEG CGM / RIGHT LEG CGM / LEFT/RIGHT STOMACH CGM KETONES NEGATIVE / TRACE / SMALL / MODERATE / LARGE
SNACK	Total Carbohydrates : ___._ grams	Carb Dose Calculation: (Meal Carbs / ___) (__._ /___) = ___.__ or __ UNITS NO INSULIN DOSE REQUIRED FOR MEALS/SNACKS UNDER __G OF CARBS OR EQUAL TO __.__ OR LESS	TIME __ : __ AM / PM LEFT ARM CGM / RIGHT ARM CGM / LEFT LEG CGM / RIGHT LEG CGM / LEFT/RIGHT STOMACH CGM KETONES NEGATIVE / TRACE / SMALL / MODERATE / LARGE
LUNCH	Total Carbohydrates : ___._ grams	Correction Dose: (BS - ___) / __ (___-___)/__ = (__/__) = ___.__ Carb Dose Calculation: (Meal Carbs / ___) (__._ /___) = ___.__ Correction Dose + Carb Dose Calculation: (___.__ + ___.__) = __.__ OR __ UNITS Correction Dose / Dose Calculation / Rounded to nearest whole number	TIME __ : __ AM / PM LEFT ARM CGM / RIGHT ARM CGM / LEFT LEG CGM / RIGHT LEG CGM / LEFT/RIGHT STOMACH CGM KETONES NEGATIVE / TRACE / SMALL / MODERATE / LARGE
SNACK	Total Carbohydrates : ___._ grams	Carb Dose Calculation: (Meal Carbs / ___) (__._ /___) = ___.__ or __ UNITS NO INSULIN DOSE REQUIRED FOR MEALS/SNACKS UNDER __G OF CARBS OR EQUAL TO __.__ OR LESS	TIME __ : __ AM / PM LEFT ARM CGM / RIGHT ARM CGM / LEFT LEG CGM / RIGHT LEG CGM / LEFT/RIGHT STOMACH CGM KETONES NEGATIVE / TRACE / SMALL / MODERATE / LARGE
DINNER	Total Carbohydrates : ___._ grams	Correction Dose: (BS - ___) / __ (___-___)/__ = (__/__) = ___.__ Carb Dose Calculation: (Meal Carbs / ___) (__._ /___) = ___.__ Correction Dose + Carb Dose Calculation: (___.__ + ___.__) = __.__ OR __ UNITS Correction Dose / Dose Calculation / Rounded to nearest whole number	TIME __ : __ AM / PM LEFT ARM CGM / RIGHT ARM CGM / LEFT LEG CGM / RIGHT LEG CGM / LEFT/RIGHT STOMACH CGM KETONES NEGATIVE / TRACE / SMALL / MODERATE / LARGE
SNACK	Total Carbohydrates : ___._ grams	Carb Dose Calculation: (Meal Carbs / ___) (__._ /___) = ___.__ or __ UNITS NO INSULIN DOSE REQUIRED FOR MEALS/SNACKS UNDER __G OF CARBS OR EQUAL TO __.__ OR LESS	TIME __ : __ AM / PM LEFT ARM CGM / RIGHT ARM CGM / LEFT LEG CGM / RIGHT LEG CGM / LEFT/RIGHT STOMACH CGM KETONES NEGATIVE / TRACE / SMALL / MODERATE / LARGE
BEDTIME __ : __ PM	BLOOD SUGAR ____ UNITS ___ LEFT ARM CGM / RIGHT ARM CGM / LEFT LEG CGM / RIGHT LEG CGM / LEFT/RIGHT STOMACH CGM KETONES NEGATIVE / TRACE / SMALL / MODERATE / LARGE	HYDRATE 2AM BLOOD SUGAR ____ ADDITIONAL BLOOD SUGAR READINGS BS ___ at __ : __ AM/PM BS ___ at __ : __ AM/PM	NOTES MEDICINE

DATE: ______________________ SUN MON TUES WED THUR FRI SAT

	MEALS AND SNACKS	CARB AND FOOD CALCULATIONS	SHOT DETAILS AND LOCATION
BREAKFAST	Total Carbohydrates : ___._ grams	Correction Dose: (BS - ___) / __ (___-___)/__ = (__/__) = ___.__ Carb Dose Calculation: (Meal Carbs / ___) (__._ /___) = ___.__ Correction Dose + Carb Dose Calculation: (__.__ + __.__) = __.__ OR __ UNITS Correction Dose / Dose Calculation / Rounded to nearest whole number	TIME __ : __ AM / PM LEFT ARM CGM / RIGHT ARM CGM / LEFT LEG CGM / RIGHT LEG CGM / LEFT/RIGHT STOMACH CGM KETONES NEGATIVE TRACE SMALL MODERATE LARGE
SNACK	Total Carbohydrates : ___._ grams	Carb Dose Calculation: (Meal Carbs / ___) (__._ /___) = ___.__ or __ UNITS NO INSULIN DOSE REQUIRED FOR MEALS/SNACKS UNDER __G OF CARBS OR EQUAL TO __.__ OR LESS	TIME __ : __ AM / PM LEFT ARM CGM / RIGHT ARM CGM / LEFT LEG CGM / RIGHT LEG CGM / LEFT/RIGHT STOMACH CGM KETONES NEGATIVE TRACE SMALL MODERATE LARGE
LUNCH	Total Carbohydrates : ___._ grams	Correction Dose: (BS - ___) / __ (___-___)/__ = (__/__) = ___.__ Carb Dose Calculation: (Meal Carbs / ___) (__._ /___) = ___.__ Correction Dose + Carb Dose Calculation: (__.__ + __.__) = __.__ OR __ UNITS Correction Dose / Dose Calculation / Rounded to nearest whole number	TIME __ : __ AM / PM LEFT ARM CGM / RIGHT ARM CGM / LEFT LEG CGM / RIGHT LEG CGM / LEFT/RIGHT STOMACH CGM KETONES NEGATIVE TRACE SMALL MODERATE LARGE
SNACK	Total Carbohydrates : ___._ grams	Carb Dose Calculation: (Meal Carbs / ___) (__._ /___) = ___.__ or __ UNITS NO INSULIN DOSE REQUIRED FOR MEALS/SNACKS UNDER __G OF CARBS OR EQUAL TO __.__ OR LESS	TIME __ : __ AM / PM LEFT ARM CGM / RIGHT ARM CGM / LEFT LEG CGM / RIGHT LEG CGM / LEFT/RIGHT STOMACH CGM KETONES NEGATIVE TRACE SMALL MODERATE LARGE
DINNER	Total Carbohydrates : ___._ grams	Correction Dose: (BS - ___) / __ (___-___)/__ = (__/__) = ___.__ Carb Dose Calculation: (Meal Carbs / ___) (__._ /___) = ___.__ Correction Dose + Carb Dose Calculation: (__.__ + __.__) = __.__ OR __ UNITS Correction Dose / Dose Calculation / Rounded to nearest whole number	TIME __ : __ AM / PM LEFT ARM CGM / RIGHT ARM CGM / LEFT LEG CGM / RIGHT LEG CGM / LEFT/RIGHT STOMACH CGM KETONES NEGATIVE TRACE SMALL MODERATE LARGE
SNACK	Total Carbohydrates : ___._ grams	Carb Dose Calculation: (Meal Carbs / ___) (__._ /___) = ___.__ or __ UNITS NO INSULIN DOSE REQUIRED FOR MEALS/SNACKS UNDER __G OF CARBS OR EQUAL TO __.__ OR LESS	TIME __ : __ AM / PM LEFT ARM CGM / RIGHT ARM CGM / LEFT LEG CGM / RIGHT LEG CGM / LEFT/RIGHT STOMACH CGM KETONES NEGATIVE TRACE SMALL MODERATE LARGE
BEDTIME __ : __ PM	BLOOD SUGAR _____ UNITS ___ LEFT ARM CGM / RIGHT ARM CGM / LEFT LEG CGM / RIGHT LEG CGM / LEFT/RIGHT STOMACH CGM KETONES NEGATIVE TRACE SMALL MODERATE LARGE	HYDRATE 2AM BLOOD SUGAR _____ ADDITIONAL BLOOD SUGAR READINGS BS ___ at __ : __ AM/PM BS ___ at __ : __ AM/PM	NOTES MEDICINE

DATE: ______________________ SUN MON TUES WED THUR FRI SAT

	MEALS AND SNACKS	CARB AND FOOD CALCULATIONS	SHOT DETAILS AND LOCATION
BREAKFAST	Total Carbohydrates : ___._ grams	Correction Dose: (BS - ___) / __ (___-___)/__ = (__/__) = ___.__ Carb Dose Calculation: (Meal Carbs / ___) (__._ /___) = ___.__ Correction Dose + Carb Dose Calculation: (_____ + _____) = __.__ OR __ UNITS Correction Dose / Dose Calculation / Rounded to nearest whole number	TIME __ : __ AM / PM LEFT ARM CGM / RIGHT ARM CGM / LEFT LEG CGM / RIGHT LEG CGM / LEFT/RIGHT STOMACH CGM KETONES NEGATIVE / TRACE / SMALL / MODERATE / LARGE
SNACK	Total Carbohydrates : ___._ grams	Carb Dose Calculation: (Meal Carbs / ___) (__._ /___) = ___.__ or __ UNITS NO INSULIN DOSE REQUIRED FOR MEALS/SNACKS UNDER __G OF CARBS OR EQUAL TO __.__ OR LESS	TIME __ : __ AM / PM LEFT ARM CGM / RIGHT ARM CGM / LEFT LEG CGM / RIGHT LEG CGM / LEFT/RIGHT STOMACH CGM KETONES NEGATIVE / TRACE / SMALL / MODERATE / LARGE
LUNCH	Total Carbohydrates : ___._ grams	Correction Dose: (BS - ___) / __ (___-___)/__ = (__/__) = ___.__ Carb Dose Calculation: (Meal Carbs / ___) (__._ /___) = ___.__ Correction Dose + Carb Dose Calculation: (_____ + _____) = __.__ OR __ UNITS Correction Dose / Dose Calculation / Rounded to nearest whole number	TIME __ : __ AM / PM LEFT ARM CGM / RIGHT ARM CGM / LEFT LEG CGM / RIGHT LEG CGM / LEFT/RIGHT STOMACH CGM KETONES NEGATIVE / TRACE / SMALL / MODERATE / LARGE
SNACK	Total Carbohydrates : ___._ grams	Carb Dose Calculation: (Meal Carbs / ___) (__._ /___) = ___.__ or __ UNITS NO INSULIN DOSE REQUIRED FOR MEALS/SNACKS UNDER __G OF CARBS OR EQUAL TO __.__ OR LESS	TIME __ : __ AM / PM LEFT ARM CGM / RIGHT ARM CGM / LEFT LEG CGM / RIGHT LEG CGM / LEFT/RIGHT STOMACH CGM KETONES NEGATIVE / TRACE / SMALL / MODERATE / LARGE
DINNER	Total Carbohydrates : ___._ grams	Correction Dose: (BS - ___) / __ (___-___)/__ = (__/__) = ___.__ Carb Dose Calculation: (Meal Carbs / ___) (__._ /___) = ___.__ Correction Dose + Carb Dose Calculation: (_____ + _____) = __.__ OR __ UNITS Correction Dose / Dose Calculation / Rounded to nearest whole number	TIME __ : __ AM / PM LEFT ARM CGM / RIGHT ARM CGM / LEFT LEG CGM / RIGHT LEG CGM / LEFT/RIGHT STOMACH CGM KETONES NEGATIVE / TRACE / SMALL / MODERATE / LARGE
SNACK	Total Carbohydrates : ___._ grams	Carb Dose Calculation: (Meal Carbs / ___) (__._ /___) = ___.__ or __ UNITS NO INSULIN DOSE REQUIRED FOR MEALS/SNACKS UNDER __G OF CARBS OR EQUAL TO __.__ OR LESS	TIME __ : __ AM / PM LEFT ARM CGM / RIGHT ARM CGM / LEFT LEG CGM / RIGHT LEG CGM / LEFT/RIGHT STOMACH CGM KETONES NEGATIVE / TRACE / SMALL / MODERATE / LARGE
BEDTIME __ : __ PM	BLOOD SUGAR ______ UNITS ___ LEFT ARM CGM / RIGHT ARM CGM / LEFT LEG CGM / RIGHT LEG CGM / LEFT/RIGHT STOMACH CGM KETONES NEGATIVE / TRACE / SMALL / MODERATE / LARGE	HYDRATE 2AM BLOOD SUGAR _____ ADDITIONAL BLOOD SUGAR READINGS BS ___ at __ : __ AM/PM BS ___ at __ : __ AM/PM	NOTES MEDICINE

DATE: ______________________________ SUN MON TUES WED THUR FRI SAT

	MEALS AND SNACKS	CARB AND FOOD CALCULATIONS	SHOT DETAILS AND LOCATION
BREAKFAST	Total Carbohydrates : ___._ grams	Correction Dose: (BS - ___) / __ (___-___)/__ = (__/__) = ___.__ Carb Dose Calculation: (Meal Carbs / ___) (__._ /___) = ___.__ Correction Dose + Carb Dose Calculation: (__.__ + __.__) = __.__ OR __ UNITS Correction Dose / Dose Calculation / Rounded to nearest whole number	TIME __ : __ AM / PM LEFT ARM CGM / RIGHT ARM CGM / LEFT LEG CGM / RIGHT LEG CGM / LEFT/RIGHT STOMACH CGM KETONES NEGATIVE / TRACE / SMALL / MODERATE / LARGE
SNACK	Total Carbohydrates : ___._ grams	Carb Dose Calculation: (Meal Carbs / ___) (__._ /___) = ___.__ or __ UNITS NO INSULIN DOSE REQUIRED FOR MEALS/SNACKS UNDER __G OF CARBS OR EQUAL TO __.__ OR LESS	TIME __ : __ AM / PM LEFT ARM CGM / RIGHT ARM CGM / LEFT LEG CGM / RIGHT LEG CGM / LEFT/RIGHT STOMACH CGM KETONES NEGATIVE / TRACE / SMALL / MODERATE / LARGE
LUNCH	Total Carbohydrates : ___._ grams	Correction Dose: (BS - ___) / __ (___-___)/__ = (__/__) = ___.__ Carb Dose Calculation: (Meal Carbs / ___) (__._ /___) = ___.__ Correction Dose + Carb Dose Calculation: (__.__ + __.__) = __.__ OR __ UNITS Correction Dose / Dose Calculation / Rounded to nearest whole number	TIME __ : __ AM / PM LEFT ARM CGM / RIGHT ARM CGM / LEFT LEG CGM / RIGHT LEG CGM / LEFT/RIGHT STOMACH CGM KETONES NEGATIVE / TRACE / SMALL / MODERATE / LARGE
SNACK	Total Carbohydrates : ___._ grams	Carb Dose Calculation: (Meal Carbs / ___) (__._ /___) = ___.__ or __ UNITS NO INSULIN DOSE REQUIRED FOR MEALS/SNACKS UNDER __G OF CARBS OR EQUAL TO __.__ OR LESS	TIME __ : __ AM / PM LEFT ARM CGM / RIGHT ARM CGM / LEFT LEG CGM / RIGHT LEG CGM / LEFT/RIGHT STOMACH CGM KETONES NEGATIVE / TRACE / SMALL / MODERATE / LARGE
DINNER	Total Carbohydrates : ___._ grams	Correction Dose: (BS - ___) / __ (___-___)/__ = (__/__) = ___.__ Carb Dose Calculation: (Meal Carbs / ___) (__._ /___) = ___.__ Correction Dose + Carb Dose Calculation: (__.__ + __.__) = __.__ OR __ UNITS Correction Dose / Dose Calculation / Rounded to nearest whole number	TIME __ : __ AM / PM LEFT ARM CGM / RIGHT ARM CGM / LEFT LEG CGM / RIGHT LEG CGM / LEFT/RIGHT STOMACH CGM KETONES NEGATIVE / TRACE / SMALL / MODERATE / LARGE
SNACK	Total Carbohydrates : ___._ grams	Carb Dose Calculation: (Meal Carbs / ___) (__._ /___) = ___.__ or __ UNITS NO INSULIN DOSE REQUIRED FOR MEALS/SNACKS UNDER __G OF CARBS OR EQUAL TO __.__ OR LESS	TIME __ : __ AM / PM LEFT ARM CGM / RIGHT ARM CGM / LEFT LEG CGM / RIGHT LEG CGM / LEFT/RIGHT STOMACH CGM KETONES NEGATIVE / TRACE / SMALL / MODERATE / LARGE
BEDTIME __ : __ PM	BLOOD SUGAR ____ UNITS ___ LEFT ARM CGM / RIGHT ARM CGM / LEFT LEG CGM / RIGHT LEG CGM / LEFT/RIGHT STOMACH CGM KETONES NEGATIVE / TRACE / SMALL / MODERATE / LARGE	HYDRATE 2AM BLOOD SUGAR _____ ADDITIONAL BLOOD SUGAR READINGS BS ___ at __ : __ AM/PM BS ___ at __ : __ AM/PM	NOTES MEDICINE

DATE: ______________________________ SUN MON TUES WED THUR FRI SAT

	MEALS AND SNACKS	CARB AND FOOD CALCULATIONS	SHOT DETAILS AND LOCATION
BREAKFAST	Total Carbohydrates : ___._ grams	Correction Dose: (BS - ___) / __ (___-___)/__ = (__/__) = ___.__ Carb Dose Calculation: (Meal Carbs / ___) (__._ /___) = ___.__ Correction Dose + Carb Dose Calculation: (__.__ + __.__) = __.__ OR __ UNITS Correction Dose / Dose Calculation / Rounded to nearest whole number	TIME __ : __ AM / PM LEFT ARM CGM / RIGHT ARM CGM / LEFT LEG CGM / RIGHT LEG CGM / LEFT/RIGHT STOMACH CGM KETONES NEGATIVE / TRACE / SMALL / MODERATE / LARGE
SNACK	Total Carbohydrates : ___._ grams	Carb Dose Calculation: (Meal Carbs / ___) (__._ /___) = ___.__ or __ UNITS NO INSULIN DOSE REQUIRED FOR MEALS/SNACKS UNDER __G OF CARBS OR EQUAL TO __.__ OR LESS	TIME __ : __ AM / PM LEFT ARM CGM / RIGHT ARM CGM / LEFT LEG CGM / RIGHT LEG CGM / LEFT/RIGHT STOMACH CGM KETONES NEGATIVE / TRACE / SMALL / MODERATE / LARGE
LUNCH	Total Carbohydrates : ___._ grams	Correction Dose: (BS - ___) / __ (___-___)/__ = (__/__) = ___.__ Carb Dose Calculation: (Meal Carbs / ___) (__._ /___) = ___.__ Correction Dose + Carb Dose Calculation: (__.__ + __.__) = __.__ OR __ UNITS Correction Dose / Dose Calculation / Rounded to nearest whole number	TIME __ : __ AM / PM LEFT ARM CGM / RIGHT ARM CGM / LEFT LEG CGM / RIGHT LEG CGM / LEFT/RIGHT STOMACH CGM KETONES NEGATIVE / TRACE / SMALL / MODERATE / LARGE
SNACK	Total Carbohydrates : ___._ grams	Carb Dose Calculation: (Meal Carbs / ___) (__._ /___) = ___.__ or __ UNITS NO INSULIN DOSE REQUIRED FOR MEALS/SNACKS UNDER __G OF CARBS OR EQUAL TO __.__ OR LESS	TIME __ : __ AM / PM LEFT ARM CGM / RIGHT ARM CGM / LEFT LEG CGM / RIGHT LEG CGM / LEFT/RIGHT STOMACH CGM KETONES NEGATIVE / TRACE / SMALL / MODERATE / LARGE
DINNER	Total Carbohydrates : ___._ grams	Correction Dose: (BS - ___) / __ (___-___)/__ = (__/__) = ___.__ Carb Dose Calculation: (Meal Carbs / ___) (__._ /___) = ___.__ Correction Dose + Carb Dose Calculation: (__.__ + __.__) = __.__ OR __ UNITS Correction Dose / Dose Calculation / Rounded to nearest whole number	TIME __ : __ AM / PM LEFT ARM CGM / RIGHT ARM CGM / LEFT LEG CGM / RIGHT LEG CGM / LEFT/RIGHT STOMACH CGM KETONES NEGATIVE / TRACE / SMALL / MODERATE / LARGE
SNACK	Total Carbohydrates : ___._ grams	Carb Dose Calculation: (Meal Carbs / ___) (__._ /___) = ___.__ or __ UNITS NO INSULIN DOSE REQUIRED FOR MEALS/SNACKS UNDER __G OF CARBS OR EQUAL TO __.__ OR LESS	TIME __ : __ AM / PM LEFT ARM CGM / RIGHT ARM CGM / LEFT LEG CGM / RIGHT LEG CGM / LEFT/RIGHT STOMACH CGM KETONES NEGATIVE / TRACE / SMALL / MODERATE / LARGE
BEDTIME __ : __ PM	BLOOD SUGAR ____ UNITS ___ LEFT ARM CGM / RIGHT ARM CGM / LEFT LEG CGM / RIGHT LEG CGM / LEFT/RIGHT STOMACH CGM KETONES NEGATIVE / TRACE / SMALL / MODERATE / LARGE	HYDRATE 2AM BLOOD SUGAR ____ ADDITIONAL BLOOD SUGAR READINGS BS ___ at __ : __ AM/PM BS ___ at __ : __ AM/PM	NOTES MEDICINE

DATE: ______________________________ SUN MON TUES WED THUR FRI SAT

	MEALS AND SNACKS	CARB AND FOOD CALCULATIONS	SHOT DETAILS AND LOCATION
BREAKFAST	Total Carbohydrates : ___._ grams	Correction Dose: (BS - ___) / __ (___-___)/__ = (__/__) = ___.__ Carb Dose Calculation: (Meal Carbs / ___) (__._ /___) = ___.__ Correction Dose + Carb Dose Calculation: (___.__ + ___.__) = __.__ OR __ UNITS Correction Dose · Dose Calculation · Rounded to nearest whole number	TIME __ : __ AM / PM LEFT ARM CGM · RIGHT ARM CGM · LEFT LEG CGM · RIGHT LEG CGM · LEFT/RIGHT STOMACH CGM KETONES NEGATIVE · TRACE · SMALL · MODERATE · LARGE
SNACK	Total Carbohydrates : ___._ grams	Carb Dose Calculation: (Meal Carbs / ___) (__._ /___) = ___.__ or __ UNITS NO INSULIN DOSE REQUIRED FOR MEALS/SNACKS UNDER __G OF CARBS OR EQUAL TO __.__ OR LESS	TIME __ : __ AM / PM LEFT ARM CGM · RIGHT ARM CGM · LEFT LEG CGM · RIGHT LEG CGM · LEFT/RIGHT STOMACH CGM KETONES NEGATIVE · TRACE · SMALL · MODERATE · LARGE
LUNCH	Total Carbohydrates : ___._ grams	Correction Dose: (BS - ___) / __ (___-___)/__ = (__/__) = ___.__ Carb Dose Calculation: (Meal Carbs / ___) (__._ /___) = ___.__ Correction Dose + Carb Dose Calculation: (___.__ + ___.__) = __.__ OR __ UNITS Correction Dose · Dose Calculation · Rounded to nearest whole number	TIME __ : __ AM / PM LEFT ARM CGM · RIGHT ARM CGM · LEFT LEG CGM · RIGHT LEG CGM · LEFT/RIGHT STOMACH CGM KETONES NEGATIVE · TRACE · SMALL · MODERATE · LARGE
SNACK	Total Carbohydrates : ___._ grams	Carb Dose Calculation: (Meal Carbs / ___) (__._ /___) = ___.__ or __ UNITS NO INSULIN DOSE REQUIRED FOR MEALS/SNACKS UNDER __G OF CARBS OR EQUAL TO __.__ OR LESS	TIME __ : __ AM / PM LEFT ARM CGM · RIGHT ARM CGM · LEFT LEG CGM · RIGHT LEG CGM · LEFT/RIGHT STOMACH CGM KETONES NEGATIVE · TRACE · SMALL · MODERATE · LARGE
DINNER	Total Carbohydrates : ___._ grams	Correction Dose: (BS - ___) / __ (___-___)/__ = (__/__) = ___.__ Carb Dose Calculation: (Meal Carbs / ___) (__._ /___) = ___.__ Correction Dose + Carb Dose Calculation: (___.__ + ___.__) = __.__ OR __ UNITS Correction Dose · Dose Calculation · Rounded to nearest whole number	TIME __ : __ AM / PM LEFT ARM CGM · RIGHT ARM CGM · LEFT LEG CGM · RIGHT LEG CGM · LEFT/RIGHT STOMACH CGM KETONES NEGATIVE · TRACE · SMALL · MODERATE · LARGE
SNACK	Total Carbohydrates : ___._ grams	Carb Dose Calculation: (Meal Carbs / ___) (__._ /___) = ___.__ or __ UNITS NO INSULIN DOSE REQUIRED FOR MEALS/SNACKS UNDER __G OF CARBS OR EQUAL TO __.__ OR LESS	TIME __ : __ AM / PM LEFT ARM CGM · RIGHT ARM CGM · LEFT LEG CGM · RIGHT LEG CGM · LEFT/RIGHT STOMACH CGM KETONES NEGATIVE · TRACE · SMALL · MODERATE · LARGE
BEDTIME __ : __ PM	BLOOD SUGAR _____ UNITS ___ LEFT ARM CGM · RIGHT ARM CGM · LEFT LEG CGM · RIGHT LEG CGM · LEFT/RIGHT STOMACH CGM KETONES NEGATIVE · TRACE · SMALL · MODERATE · LARGE	HYDRATE 2AM BLOOD SUGAR _____ ADDITIONAL BLOOD SUGAR READINGS BS ___ at __ : __ AM/PM BS ___ at __ : __ AM/PM	NOTES MEDICINE

DATE: ________________________ SUN MON TUES WED THUR FRI SAT

	MEALS AND SNACKS	CARB AND FOOD CALCULATIONS	SHOT DETAILS AND LOCATION
BREAKFAST	Total Carbohydrates : ___._ grams	Correction Dose: (BS - ___) / __ (___-___)/__ = (__/__) = ___.__ Carb Dose Calculation: (Meal Carbs / ___) (__._ /___) = ___.__ Correction Dose + Carb Dose Calculation: (______ + ______) = __.__ OR __ UNITS Correction Dose / Dose Calculation / Rounded to nearest whole number	TIME __:__ AM / PM LEFT ARM CGM / RIGHT ARM CGM / LEFT LEG CGM / RIGHT LEG CGM / LEFT/RIGHT STOMACH CGM KETONES NEGATIVE TRACE SMALL MODERATE LARGE
SNACK	Total Carbohydrates : ___._ grams	Carb Dose Calculation: (Meal Carbs / ___) (__._ /___) = ___.__ or __ UNITS NO INSULIN DOSE REQUIRED FOR MEALS/SNACKS UNDER __G OF CARBS OR EQUAL TO __.__ OR LESS	TIME __:__ AM / PM LEFT ARM CGM / RIGHT ARM CGM / LEFT LEG CGM / RIGHT LEG CGM / LEFT/RIGHT STOMACH CGM KETONES NEGATIVE TRACE SMALL MODERATE LARGE
LUNCH	Total Carbohydrates : ___._ grams	Correction Dose: (BS - ___) / __ (___-___)/__ = (__/__) = ___.__ Carb Dose Calculation: (Meal Carbs / ___) (__._ /___) = ___.__ Correction Dose + Carb Dose Calculation: (______ + ______) = __.__ OR __ UNITS Correction Dose / Dose Calculation / Rounded to nearest whole number	TIME __:__ AM / PM LEFT ARM CGM / RIGHT ARM CGM / LEFT LEG CGM / RIGHT LEG CGM / LEFT/RIGHT STOMACH CGM KETONES NEGATIVE TRACE SMALL MODERATE LARGE
SNACK	Total Carbohydrates : ___._ grams	Carb Dose Calculation: (Meal Carbs / ___) (__._ /___) = ___.__ or __ UNITS NO INSULIN DOSE REQUIRED FOR MEALS/SNACKS UNDER __G OF CARBS OR EQUAL TO __.__ OR LESS	TIME __:__ AM / PM LEFT ARM CGM / RIGHT ARM CGM / LEFT LEG CGM / RIGHT LEG CGM / LEFT/RIGHT STOMACH CGM KETONES NEGATIVE TRACE SMALL MODERATE LARGE
DINNER	Total Carbohydrates : ___._ grams	Correction Dose: (BS - ___) / __ (___-___)/__ = (__/__) = ___.__ Carb Dose Calculation: (Meal Carbs / ___) (__._ /___) = ___.__ Correction Dose + Carb Dose Calculation: (______ + ______) = __.__ OR __ UNITS Correction Dose / Dose Calculation / Rounded to nearest whole number	TIME __:__ AM / PM LEFT ARM CGM / RIGHT ARM CGM / LEFT LEG CGM / RIGHT LEG CGM / LEFT/RIGHT STOMACH CGM KETONES NEGATIVE TRACE SMALL MODERATE LARGE
SNACK	Total Carbohydrates : ___._ grams	Carb Dose Calculation: (Meal Carbs / ___) (__._ /___) = ___.__ or __ UNITS NO INSULIN DOSE REQUIRED FOR MEALS/SNACKS UNDER __G OF CARBS OR EQUAL TO __.__ OR LESS	TIME __:__ AM / PM LEFT ARM CGM / RIGHT ARM CGM / LEFT LEG CGM / RIGHT LEG CGM / LEFT/RIGHT STOMACH CGM KETONES NEGATIVE TRACE SMALL MODERATE LARGE
BEDTIME __:__ PM	BLOOD SUGAR _____ UNITS ___ LEFT ARM CGM / RIGHT ARM CGM / LEFT LEG CGM / RIGHT LEG CGM / LEFT/RIGHT STOMACH CGM KETONES NEGATIVE TRACE SMALL MODERATE LARGE	HYDRATE 2AM BLOOD SUGAR _____ ADDITIONAL BLOOD SUGAR READINGS BS ___ at __ : __ AM/PM BS ___ at __ : __ AM/PM	NOTES MEDICINE

DATE: ______________________________ SUN MON TUES WED THUR FRI SAT

	MEALS AND SNACKS	CARB AND FOOD CALCULATIONS	SHOT DETAILS AND LOCATION
BREAKFAST	Total Carbohydrates : ___._ grams	Correction Dose: (BS - ___) / __ (___-___)/__ = (__/__) = ___.__ Carb Dose Calculation: (Meal Carbs / ___) (__._ /___) = ___.__ Correction Dose + Carb Dose Calculation: (___.__ + ___.__) = __.__ OR __ UNITS Correction Dose / Dose Calculation / Rounded to nearest whole number	TIME __ : __ AM / PM LEFT ARM CGM / RIGHT ARM CGM / LEFT LEG CGM / RIGHT LEG CGM / LEFT/RIGHT STOMACH CGM KETONES NEGATIVE / TRACE / SMALL / MODERATE / LARGE
SNACK	Total Carbohydrates : ___._ grams	Carb Dose Calculation: (Meal Carbs / ___) (__._ /___) = ___.__ or __ UNITS NO INSULIN DOSE REQUIRED FOR MEALS/SNACKS UNDER __G OF CARBS OR EQUAL TO __.__ OR LESS	TIME __ : __ AM / PM LEFT ARM CGM / RIGHT ARM CGM / LEFT LEG CGM / RIGHT LEG CGM / LEFT/RIGHT STOMACH CGM KETONES NEGATIVE / TRACE / SMALL / MODERATE / LARGE
LUNCH	Total Carbohydrates : ___._ grams	Correction Dose: (BS - ___) / __ (___-___)/__ = (__/__) = ___.__ Carb Dose Calculation: (Meal Carbs / ___) (__._ /___) = ___.__ Correction Dose + Carb Dose Calculation: (___.__ + ___.__) = __.__ OR __ UNITS Correction Dose / Dose Calculation / Rounded to nearest whole number	TIME __ : __ AM / PM LEFT ARM CGM / RIGHT ARM CGM / LEFT LEG CGM / RIGHT LEG CGM / LEFT/RIGHT STOMACH CGM KETONES NEGATIVE / TRACE / SMALL / MODERATE / LARGE
SNACK	Total Carbohydrates : ___._ grams	Carb Dose Calculation: (Meal Carbs / ___) (__._ /___) = ___.__ or __ UNITS NO INSULIN DOSE REQUIRED FOR MEALS/SNACKS UNDER __G OF CARBS OR EQUAL TO __.__ OR LESS	TIME __ : __ AM / PM LEFT ARM CGM / RIGHT ARM CGM / LEFT LEG CGM / RIGHT LEG CGM / LEFT/RIGHT STOMACH CGM KETONES NEGATIVE / TRACE / SMALL / MODERATE / LARGE
DINNER	Total Carbohydrates : ___._ grams	Correction Dose: (BS - ___) / __ (___-___)/__ = (__/__) = ___.__ Carb Dose Calculation: (Meal Carbs / ___) (__._ /___) = ___.__ Correction Dose + Carb Dose Calculation: (___.__ + ___.__) = __.__ OR __ UNITS Correction Dose / Dose Calculation / Rounded to nearest whole number	TIME __ : __ AM / PM LEFT ARM CGM / RIGHT ARM CGM / LEFT LEG CGM / RIGHT LEG CGM / LEFT/RIGHT STOMACH CGM KETONES NEGATIVE / TRACE / SMALL / MODERATE / LARGE
SNACK	Total Carbohydrates : ___._ grams	Carb Dose Calculation: (Meal Carbs / ___) (__._ /___) = ___.__ or __ UNITS NO INSULIN DOSE REQUIRED FOR MEALS/SNACKS UNDER __G OF CARBS OR EQUAL TO __.__ OR LESS	TIME __ : __ AM / PM LEFT ARM CGM / RIGHT ARM CGM / LEFT LEG CGM / RIGHT LEG CGM / LEFT/RIGHT STOMACH CGM KETONES NEGATIVE / TRACE / SMALL / MODERATE / LARGE
BEDTIME __ : __ PM	BLOOD SUGAR _____ UNITS ___ LEFT ARM CGM / RIGHT ARM CGM / LEFT LEG CGM / RIGHT LEG CGM / LEFT/RIGHT STOMACH CGM KETONES NEGATIVE / TRACE / SMALL / MODERATE / LARGE	HYDRATE 2AM BLOOD SUGAR _____ ADDITIONAL BLOOD SUGAR READINGS BS ___ at __ : __ AM/PM BS ___ at __ : __ AM/PM	NOTES MEDICINE

DATE: ______________________ SUN MON TUES WED THUR FRI SAT

	MEALS AND SNACKS	CARB AND FOOD CALCULATIONS	SHOT DETAILS AND LOCATION
BREAKFAST	Total Carbohydrates : ___._ grams	Correction Dose: (BS - ___) / __ (___-___)/__ = (__/__) = ___.__ Carb Dose Calculation: (Meal Carbs / ___) (__._ /___) = ___.__ Correction Dose + Carb Dose Calculation: (____._ + ____._) = __.__ OR __ UNITS Correction Dose · Dose Calculation · Rounded to nearest whole number	TIME __ : __ AM / PM LEFT ARM CGM · RIGHT ARM CGM · LEFT LEG CGM · RIGHT LEG CGM · LEFT/RIGHT STOMACH CGM KETONES NEGATIVE · TRACE · SMALL · MODERATE · LARGE
SNACK	Total Carbohydrates : ___._ grams	Carb Dose Calculation: (Meal Carbs / ___) (__._ /___) = ___.__ or __ UNITS NO INSULIN DOSE REQUIRED FOR MEALS/SNACKS UNDER __G OF CARBS OR EQUAL TO __.__ OR LESS	TIME __ : __ AM / PM LEFT ARM CGM · RIGHT ARM CGM · LEFT LEG CGM · RIGHT LEG CGM · LEFT/RIGHT STOMACH CGM KETONES NEGATIVE · TRACE · SMALL · MODERATE · LARGE
LUNCH	Total Carbohydrates : ___._ grams	Correction Dose: (BS - ___) / __ (___-___)/__ = (__/__) = ___.__ Carb Dose Calculation: (Meal Carbs / ___) (__._ /___) = ___.__ Correction Dose + Carb Dose Calculation: (____._ + ____._) = __.__ OR __ UNITS Correction Dose · Dose Calculation · Rounded to nearest whole number	TIME __ : __ AM / PM LEFT ARM CGM · RIGHT ARM CGM · LEFT LEG CGM · RIGHT LEG CGM · LEFT/RIGHT STOMACH CGM KETONES NEGATIVE · TRACE · SMALL · MODERATE · LARGE
SNACK	Total Carbohydrates : ___._ grams	Carb Dose Calculation: (Meal Carbs / ___) (__._ /___) = ___.__ or __ UNITS NO INSULIN DOSE REQUIRED FOR MEALS/SNACKS UNDER __G OF CARBS OR EQUAL TO __.__ OR LESS	TIME __ : __ AM / PM LEFT ARM CGM · RIGHT ARM CGM · LEFT LEG CGM · RIGHT LEG CGM · LEFT/RIGHT STOMACH CGM KETONES NEGATIVE · TRACE · SMALL · MODERATE · LARGE
DINNER	Total Carbohydrates : ___._ grams	Correction Dose: (BS - ___) / __ (___-___)/__ = (__/__) = ___.__ Carb Dose Calculation: (Meal Carbs / ___) (__._ /___) = ___.__ Correction Dose + Carb Dose Calculation: (____._ + ____._) = __.__ OR __ UNITS Correction Dose · Dose Calculation · Rounded to nearest whole number	TIME __ : __ AM / PM LEFT ARM CGM · RIGHT ARM CGM · LEFT LEG CGM · RIGHT LEG CGM · LEFT/RIGHT STOMACH CGM KETONES NEGATIVE · TRACE · SMALL · MODERATE · LARGE
SNACK	Total Carbohydrates : ___._ grams	Carb Dose Calculation: (Meal Carbs / ___) (__._ /___) = ___.__ or __ UNITS NO INSULIN DOSE REQUIRED FOR MEALS/SNACKS UNDER __G OF CARBS OR EQUAL TO __.__ OR LESS	TIME __ : __ AM / PM LEFT ARM CGM · RIGHT ARM CGM · LEFT LEG CGM · RIGHT LEG CGM · LEFT/RIGHT STOMACH CGM KETONES NEGATIVE · TRACE · SMALL · MODERATE · LARGE
BEDTIME __ : __ PM	BLOOD SUGAR ____ UNITS __ LEFT ARM CGM · RIGHT ARM CGM · LEFT LEG CGM · RIGHT LEG CGM · LEFT/RIGHT STOMACH CGM KETONES NEGATIVE · TRACE · SMALL · MODERATE · LARGE	HYDRATE 2AM BLOOD SUGAR ____ ADDITIONAL BLOOD SUGAR READINGS BS ___ at __ : __ AM/PM BS ___ at __ : __ AM/PM	NOTES MEDICINE

DATE: ______________________ SUN MON TUES WED THUR FRI SAT

	MEALS AND SNACKS	CARB AND FOOD CALCULATIONS	SHOT DETAILS AND LOCATION
BREAKFAST	Total Carbohydrates : ___._ grams	Correction Dose: (BS - ___) / __ (___-___)/__ = (__/__) = ___.__ Carb Dose Calculation: (Meal Carbs / ___) (__._ /___) = ___.__ Correction Dose + Carb Dose Calculation: (_____ + _____) = __.__ OR __ UNITS Correction Dose Dose Calculation Rounded to nearest whole number	TIME __ : __ AM / PM LEFT ARM CGM, RIGHT ARM CGM, LEFT LEG CGM, RIGHT LEG CGM, LEFT/RIGHT STOMACH CGM KETONES NEGATIVE TRACE SMALL MODERATE LARGE
SNACK	Total Carbohydrates : ___._ grams	Carb Dose Calculation: (Meal Carbs / ___) (__._ /___) = ___.__ or __ UNITS NO INSULIN DOSE REQUIRED FOR MEALS/SNACKS UNDER __G OF CARBS OR EQUAL TO __.__ OR LESS	TIME __ : __ AM / PM LEFT ARM CGM, RIGHT ARM CGM, LEFT LEG CGM, RIGHT LEG CGM, LEFT/RIGHT STOMACH CGM KETONES NEGATIVE TRACE SMALL MODERATE LARGE
LUNCH	Total Carbohydrates : ___._ grams	Correction Dose: (BS - ___) / __ (___-___)/__ = (__/__) = ___.__ Carb Dose Calculation: (Meal Carbs / ___) (__._ /___) = ___.__ Correction Dose + Carb Dose Calculation: (_____ + _____) = __.__ OR __ UNITS Correction Dose Dose Calculation Rounded to nearest whole number	TIME __ : __ AM / PM LEFT ARM CGM, RIGHT ARM CGM, LEFT LEG CGM, RIGHT LEG CGM, LEFT/RIGHT STOMACH CGM KETONES NEGATIVE TRACE SMALL MODERATE LARGE
SNACK	Total Carbohydrates : ___._ grams	Carb Dose Calculation: (Meal Carbs / ___) (__._ /___) = ___.__ or __ UNITS NO INSULIN DOSE REQUIRED FOR MEALS/SNACKS UNDER __G OF CARBS OR EQUAL TO __.__ OR LESS	TIME __ : __ AM / PM LEFT ARM CGM, RIGHT ARM CGM, LEFT LEG CGM, RIGHT LEG CGM, LEFT/RIGHT STOMACH CGM KETONES NEGATIVE TRACE SMALL MODERATE LARGE
DINNER	Total Carbohydrates : ___._ grams	Correction Dose: (BS - ___) / __ (___-___)/__ = (__/__) = ___.__ Carb Dose Calculation: (Meal Carbs / ___) (__._ /___) = ___.__ Correction Dose + Carb Dose Calculation: (_____ + _____) = __.__ OR __ UNITS Correction Dose Dose Calculation Rounded to nearest whole number	TIME __ : __ AM / PM LEFT ARM CGM, RIGHT ARM CGM, LEFT LEG CGM, RIGHT LEG CGM, LEFT/RIGHT STOMACH CGM KETONES NEGATIVE TRACE SMALL MODERATE LARGE
SNACK	Total Carbohydrates : ___._ grams	Carb Dose Calculation: (Meal Carbs / ___) (__._ /___) = ___.__ or __ UNITS NO INSULIN DOSE REQUIRED FOR MEALS/SNACKS UNDER __G OF CARBS OR EQUAL TO __.__ OR LESS	TIME __ : __ AM / PM LEFT ARM CGM, RIGHT ARM CGM, LEFT LEG CGM, RIGHT LEG CGM, LEFT/RIGHT STOMACH CGM KETONES NEGATIVE TRACE SMALL MODERATE LARGE
BEDTIME __ : __ PM	BLOOD SUGAR _____ UNITS ___ LEFT ARM CGM, RIGHT ARM CGM, LEFT LEG CGM, RIGHT LEG CGM, LEFT/RIGHT STOMACH CGM KETONES NEGATIVE TRACE SMALL MODERATE LARGE	HYDRATE 2AM BLOOD SUGAR _____ ADDITIONAL BLOOD SUGAR READINGS BS ___ at __ : __ AM/PM BS ___ at __ : __ AM/PM	NOTES MEDICINE

DATE: ______________________ SUN MON TUES WED THUR FRI SAT

	MEALS AND SNACKS	CARB AND FOOD CALCULATIONS	SHOT DETAILS AND LOCATION
BREAKFAST	Total Carbohydrates : ___._ grams	Correction Dose: (BS - ___) / __ (___-___)/__ = (__/__) = ___.__ Carb Dose Calculation: (Meal Carbs / ___) (__._ /___) = ___.__ Correction Dose + Carb Dose Calculation: (__.__ + __.__) = __.__ OR __ UNITS Correction Dose / Dose Calculation / Rounded to nearest whole number	TIME __ : __ AM / PM LEFT ARM CGM / RIGHT ARM CGM / LEFT LEG CGM / RIGHT LEG CGM / LEFT/RIGHT STOMACH CGM KETONES NEGATIVE / TRACE / SMALL / MODERATE / LARGE
SNACK	Total Carbohydrates : ___._ grams	Carb Dose Calculation: (Meal Carbs / ___) (__._ /___) = ___.__ or __ UNITS NO INSULIN DOSE REQUIRED FOR MEALS/SNACKS UNDER __G OF CARBS OR EQUAL TO __.__ OR LESS	TIME __ : __ AM / PM LEFT ARM CGM / RIGHT ARM CGM / LEFT LEG CGM / RIGHT LEG CGM / LEFT/RIGHT STOMACH CGM KETONES NEGATIVE / TRACE / SMALL / MODERATE / LARGE
LUNCH	Total Carbohydrates : ___._ grams	Correction Dose: (BS - ___) / __ (___-___)/__ = (__/__) = ___.__ Carb Dose Calculation: (Meal Carbs / ___) (__._ /___) = ___.__ Correction Dose + Carb Dose Calculation: (__.__ + __.__) = __.__ OR __ UNITS Correction Dose / Dose Calculation / Rounded to nearest whole number	TIME __ : __ AM / PM LEFT ARM CGM / RIGHT ARM CGM / LEFT LEG CGM / RIGHT LEG CGM / LEFT/RIGHT STOMACH CGM KETONES NEGATIVE / TRACE / SMALL / MODERATE / LARGE
SNACK	Total Carbohydrates : ___._ grams	Carb Dose Calculation: (Meal Carbs / ___) (__._ /___) = ___.__ or __ UNITS NO INSULIN DOSE REQUIRED FOR MEALS/SNACKS UNDER __G OF CARBS OR EQUAL TO __.__ OR LESS	TIME __ : __ AM / PM LEFT ARM CGM / RIGHT ARM CGM / LEFT LEG CGM / RIGHT LEG CGM / LEFT/RIGHT STOMACH CGM KETONES NEGATIVE / TRACE / SMALL / MODERATE / LARGE
DINNER	Total Carbohydrates : ___._ grams	Correction Dose: (BS - ___) / __ (___-___)/__ = (__/__) = ___.__ Carb Dose Calculation: (Meal Carbs / ___) (__._ /___) = ___.__ Correction Dose + Carb Dose Calculation: (__.__ + __.__) = __.__ OR __ UNITS Correction Dose / Dose Calculation / Rounded to nearest whole number	TIME __ : __ AM / PM LEFT ARM CGM / RIGHT ARM CGM / LEFT LEG CGM / RIGHT LEG CGM / LEFT/RIGHT STOMACH CGM KETONES NEGATIVE / TRACE / SMALL / MODERATE / LARGE
SNACK	Total Carbohydrates : ___._ grams	Carb Dose Calculation: (Meal Carbs / ___) (__._ /___) = ___.__ or __ UNITS NO INSULIN DOSE REQUIRED FOR MEALS/SNACKS UNDER __G OF CARBS OR EQUAL TO __.__ OR LESS	TIME __ : __ AM / PM LEFT ARM CGM / RIGHT ARM CGM / LEFT LEG CGM / RIGHT LEG CGM / LEFT/RIGHT STOMACH CGM KETONES NEGATIVE / TRACE / SMALL / MODERATE / LARGE
BEDTIME __ : __ PM	BLOOD SUGAR _____ UNITS ___ LEFT ARM CGM / RIGHT ARM CGM / LEFT LEG CGM / RIGHT LEG CGM / LEFT/RIGHT STOMACH CGM KETONES NEGATIVE / TRACE / SMALL / MODERATE / LARGE	HYDRATE 2AM BLOOD SUGAR _____ ADDITIONAL BLOOD SUGAR READINGS BS ___ at __ : __ AM/PM BS ___ at __ : __ AM/PM	NOTES MEDICINE

DATE: ____________________ SUN MON TUES WED THUR FRI SAT

	MEALS AND SNACKS	CARB AND FOOD CALCULATIONS	SHOT DETAILS AND LOCATION
BREAKFAST	Total Carbohydrates : ___._ grams	Correction Dose: (BS - ___) / __ (___-___)/__ = (__/__) = ___.__ Carb Dose Calculation: (Meal Carbs / ___) (__._ /___) = ___.__ Correction Dose + Carb Dose Calculation: (___.__ + ___.__) = __.__ OR __ UNITS Correction Dose / Dose Calculation / Rounded to nearest whole number	TIME __ : __ AM / PM LEFT ARM CGM / RIGHT ARM CGM / LEFT LEG CGM / RIGHT LEG CGM / LEFT/RIGHT STOMACH CGM KETONES NEGATIVE / TRACE / SMALL / MODERATE / LARGE
SNACK	Total Carbohydrates : ___._ grams	Carb Dose Calculation: (Meal Carbs / ___) (__._ /___) = ___.__ or __ UNITS NO INSULIN DOSE REQUIRED FOR MEALS/SNACKS UNDER __G OF CARBS OR EQUAL TO __.__ OR LESS	TIME __ : __ AM / PM LEFT ARM CGM / RIGHT ARM CGM / LEFT LEG CGM / RIGHT LEG CGM / LEFT/RIGHT STOMACH CGM KETONES NEGATIVE / TRACE / SMALL / MODERATE / LARGE
LUNCH	Total Carbohydrates : ___._ grams	Correction Dose: (BS - ___) / __ (___-___)/__ = (__/__) = ___.__ Carb Dose Calculation: (Meal Carbs / ___) (__._ /___) = ___.__ Correction Dose + Carb Dose Calculation: (___.__ + ___.__) = __.__ OR __ UNITS Correction Dose / Dose Calculation / Rounded to nearest whole number	TIME __ : __ AM / PM LEFT ARM CGM / RIGHT ARM CGM / LEFT LEG CGM / RIGHT LEG CGM / LEFT/RIGHT STOMACH CGM KETONES NEGATIVE / TRACE / SMALL / MODERATE / LARGE
SNACK	Total Carbohydrates : ___._ grams	Carb Dose Calculation: (Meal Carbs / ___) (__._ /___) = ___.__ or __ UNITS NO INSULIN DOSE REQUIRED FOR MEALS/SNACKS UNDER __G OF CARBS OR EQUAL TO __.__ OR LESS	TIME __ : __ AM / PM LEFT ARM CGM / RIGHT ARM CGM / LEFT LEG CGM / RIGHT LEG CGM / LEFT/RIGHT STOMACH CGM KETONES NEGATIVE / TRACE / SMALL / MODERATE / LARGE
DINNER	Total Carbohydrates : ___._ grams	Correction Dose: (BS - ___) / __ (___-___)/__ = (__/__) = ___.__ Carb Dose Calculation: (Meal Carbs / ___) (__._ /___) = ___.__ Correction Dose + Carb Dose Calculation: (___.__ + ___.__) = __.__ OR __ UNITS Correction Dose / Dose Calculation / Rounded to nearest whole number	TIME __ : __ AM / PM LEFT ARM CGM / RIGHT ARM CGM / LEFT LEG CGM / RIGHT LEG CGM / LEFT/RIGHT STOMACH CGM KETONES NEGATIVE / TRACE / SMALL / MODERATE / LARGE
SNACK	Total Carbohydrates : ___._ grams	Carb Dose Calculation: (Meal Carbs / ___) (__._ /___) = ___.__ or __ UNITS NO INSULIN DOSE REQUIRED FOR MEALS/SNACKS UNDER __G OF CARBS OR EQUAL TO __.__ OR LESS	TIME __ : __ AM / PM LEFT ARM CGM / RIGHT ARM CGM / LEFT LEG CGM / RIGHT LEG CGM / LEFT/RIGHT STOMACH CGM KETONES NEGATIVE / TRACE / SMALL / MODERATE / LARGE
BEDTIME __ : __ PM	BLOOD SUGAR ____ UNITS ___ LEFT ARM CGM / RIGHT ARM CGM / LEFT LEG CGM / RIGHT LEG CGM / LEFT/RIGHT STOMACH CGM KETONES NEGATIVE / TRACE / SMALL / MODERATE / LARGE	HYDRATE 2AM BLOOD SUGAR ____ ADDITIONAL BLOOD SUGAR READINGS BS ___ at __ : __ AM/PM BS ___ at __ : __ AM/PM	NOTES MEDICINE

DATE: ______________________________ SUN MON TUES WED THUR FRI SAT

	MEALS AND SNACKS	CARB AND FOOD CALCULATIONS	SHOT DETAILS AND LOCATION
BREAKFAST	Total Carbohydrates : ___._ grams	Correction Dose: (BS - ___) / __ (___-___)/__ = (__/__) = ___.__ Carb Dose Calculation: (Meal Carbs / ___) (__._ /___) = ___.__ Correction Dose + Carb Dose Calculation: (_____ + _____) = __.__ OR __ UNITS Correction Dose / Dose Calculation / Rounded to nearest whole number	TIME __ : __ AM / PM LEFT ARM CGM / RIGHT ARM CGM / LEFT LEG CGM / RIGHT LEG CGM / LEFT/RIGHT STOMACH CGM KETONES NEGATIVE / TRACE / SMALL / MODERATE / LARGE
SNACK	Total Carbohydrates : ___._ grams	Carb Dose Calculation: (Meal Carbs / ___) (__._ /___) = ___.__ or __ UNITS NO INSULIN DOSE REQUIRED FOR MEALS/SNACKS UNDER __G OF CARBS OR EQUAL TO __.__ OR LESS	TIME __ : __ AM / PM LEFT ARM CGM / RIGHT ARM CGM / LEFT LEG CGM / RIGHT LEG CGM / LEFT/RIGHT STOMACH CGM KETONES NEGATIVE / TRACE / SMALL / MODERATE / LARGE
LUNCH	Total Carbohydrates : ___._ grams	Correction Dose: (BS - ___) / __ (___-___)/__ = (__/__) = ___.__ Carb Dose Calculation: (Meal Carbs / ___) (__._ /___) = ___.__ Correction Dose + Carb Dose Calculation: (_____ + _____) = __.__ OR __ UNITS Correction Dose / Dose Calculation / Rounded to nearest whole number	TIME __ : __ AM / PM LEFT ARM CGM / RIGHT ARM CGM / LEFT LEG CGM / RIGHT LEG CGM / LEFT/RIGHT STOMACH CGM KETONES NEGATIVE / TRACE / SMALL / MODERATE / LARGE
SNACK	Total Carbohydrates : ___._ grams	Carb Dose Calculation: (Meal Carbs / ___) (__._ /___) = ___.__ or __ UNITS NO INSULIN DOSE REQUIRED FOR MEALS/SNACKS UNDER __G OF CARBS OR EQUAL TO __.__ OR LESS	TIME __ : __ AM / PM LEFT ARM CGM / RIGHT ARM CGM / LEFT LEG CGM / RIGHT LEG CGM / LEFT/RIGHT STOMACH CGM KETONES NEGATIVE / TRACE / SMALL / MODERATE / LARGE
DINNER	Total Carbohydrates : ___._ grams	Correction Dose: (BS - ___) / __ (___-___)/__ = (__/__) = ___.__ Carb Dose Calculation: (Meal Carbs / ___) (__._ /___) = ___.__ Correction Dose + Carb Dose Calculation: (_____ + _____) = __.__ OR __ UNITS Correction Dose / Dose Calculation / Rounded to nearest whole number	TIME __ : __ AM / PM LEFT ARM CGM / RIGHT ARM CGM / LEFT LEG CGM / RIGHT LEG CGM / LEFT/RIGHT STOMACH CGM KETONES NEGATIVE / TRACE / SMALL / MODERATE / LARGE
SNACK	Total Carbohydrates : ___._ grams	Carb Dose Calculation: (Meal Carbs / ___) (__._ /___) = ___.__ or __ UNITS NO INSULIN DOSE REQUIRED FOR MEALS/SNACKS UNDER __G OF CARBS OR EQUAL TO __.__ OR LESS	TIME __ : __ AM / PM LEFT ARM CGM / RIGHT ARM CGM / LEFT LEG CGM / RIGHT LEG CGM / LEFT/RIGHT STOMACH CGM KETONES NEGATIVE / TRACE / SMALL / MODERATE / LARGE
BEDTIME __ : __ PM	BLOOD SUGAR ____ UNITS ___ LEFT ARM CGM / RIGHT ARM CGM / LEFT LEG CGM / RIGHT LEG CGM / LEFT/RIGHT STOMACH CGM KETONES NEGATIVE / TRACE / SMALL / MODERATE / LARGE	HYDRATE 2AM BLOOD SUGAR ____ ADDITIONAL BLOOD SUGAR READINGS BS ___ at __ : __ AM/PM BS ___ at __ : __ AM/PM	NOTES MEDICINE

DATE: ____________________

SUN MON TUES WED THUR FRI SAT

	MEALS AND SNACKS	CARB AND FOOD CALCULATIONS	SHOT DETAILS AND LOCATION
BREAKFAST	Total Carbohydrates : ___._ grams	Correction Dose: (BS - ___) / __ (___-___)/__ = (__/__) = ___.__ Carb Dose Calculation: (Meal Carbs / ___) (__._ /___) = ___.__ Correction Dose + Carb Dose Calculation: (_____ + _____) = __.__ OR __ UNITS Correction Dose / Dose Calculation / Rounded to nearest whole number	TIME __ : __ AM / PM LEFT ARM CGM / RIGHT ARM CGM / LEFT LEG CGM / RIGHT LEG CGM / LEFT/RIGHT STOMACH CGM KETONES NEGATIVE / TRACE / SMALL / MODERATE / LARGE
SNACK	Total Carbohydrates : ___._ grams	Carb Dose Calculation: (Meal Carbs / ___) (__._ /___) = ___.__ or __ UNITS NO INSULIN DOSE REQUIRED FOR MEALS/SNACKS UNDER __G OF CARBS OR EQUAL TO __.__ OR LESS	TIME __ : __ AM / PM LEFT ARM CGM / RIGHT ARM CGM / LEFT LEG CGM / RIGHT LEG CGM / LEFT/RIGHT STOMACH CGM KETONES NEGATIVE / TRACE / SMALL / MODERATE / LARGE
LUNCH	Total Carbohydrates : ___._ grams	Correction Dose: (BS - ___) / __ (___-___)/__ = (__/__) = ___.__ Carb Dose Calculation: (Meal Carbs / ___) (__._ /___) = ___.__ Correction Dose + Carb Dose Calculation: (_____ + _____) = __.__ OR __ UNITS Correction Dose / Dose Calculation / Rounded to nearest whole number	TIME __ : __ AM / PM LEFT ARM CGM / RIGHT ARM CGM / LEFT LEG CGM / RIGHT LEG CGM / LEFT/RIGHT STOMACH CGM KETONES NEGATIVE / TRACE / SMALL / MODERATE / LARGE
SNACK	Total Carbohydrates : ___._ grams	Carb Dose Calculation: (Meal Carbs / ___) (__._ /___) = ___.__ or __ UNITS NO INSULIN DOSE REQUIRED FOR MEALS/SNACKS UNDER __G OF CARBS OR EQUAL TO __.__ OR LESS	TIME __ : __ AM / PM LEFT ARM CGM / RIGHT ARM CGM / LEFT LEG CGM / RIGHT LEG CGM / LEFT/RIGHT STOMACH CGM KETONES NEGATIVE / TRACE / SMALL / MODERATE / LARGE
DINNER	Total Carbohydrates : ___._ grams	Correction Dose: (BS - ___) / __ (___-___)/__ = (__/__) = ___.__ Carb Dose Calculation: (Meal Carbs / ___) (__._ /___) = ___.__ Correction Dose + Carb Dose Calculation: (_____ + _____) = __.__ OR __ UNITS Correction Dose / Dose Calculation / Rounded to nearest whole number	TIME __ : __ AM / PM LEFT ARM CGM / RIGHT ARM CGM / LEFT LEG CGM / RIGHT LEG CGM / LEFT/RIGHT STOMACH CGM KETONES NEGATIVE / TRACE / SMALL / MODERATE / LARGE
SNACK	Total Carbohydrates : ___._ grams	Carb Dose Calculation: (Meal Carbs / ___) (__._ /___) = ___.__ or __ UNITS NO INSULIN DOSE REQUIRED FOR MEALS/SNACKS UNDER __G OF CARBS OR EQUAL TO __.__ OR LESS	TIME __ : __ AM / PM LEFT ARM CGM / RIGHT ARM CGM / LEFT LEG CGM / RIGHT LEG CGM / LEFT/RIGHT STOMACH CGM KETONES NEGATIVE / TRACE / SMALL / MODERATE / LARGE
BEDTIME __ : __ PM	BLOOD SUGAR _____ UNITS ___ LEFT ARM CGM / RIGHT ARM CGM / LEFT LEG CGM / RIGHT LEG CGM / LEFT/RIGHT STOMACH CGM KETONES NEGATIVE / TRACE / SMALL / MODERATE / LARGE	HYDRATE 2AM BLOOD SUGAR _____ ADDITIONAL BLOOD SUGAR READINGS BS ___ at __ : __ AM/PM BS ___ at __ : __ AM/PM	NOTES MEDICINE

DATE: ______________________ SUN MON TUES WED THUR FRI SAT

	MEALS AND SNACKS	CARB AND FOOD CALCULATIONS	SHOT DETAILS AND LOCATION
BREAKFAST	Total Carbohydrates : ___._ grams	Correction Dose: (BS - ___) / __ (___-___)/__ = (__/__) = ___.__ Carb Dose Calculation: (Meal Carbs / ___) (__._ /___) = ___.__ Correction Dose + Carb Dose Calculation: (___.__ + ___.__) = __.__ OR __ UNITS Correction Dose / Dose Calculation / Rounded to nearest whole number	TIME __ : __ AM / PM LEFT ARM (CGM) / RIGHT ARM (CGM) / LEFT LEG (CGM) / RIGHT LEG (CGM) / LEFT/RIGHT STOMACH (CGM) KETONES NEGATIVE / TRACE / SMALL / MODERATE / LARGE
SNACK	Total Carbohydrates : ___._ grams	Carb Dose Calculation: (Meal Carbs / ___) (__._ /___) = ___.__ or __ UNITS NO INSULIN DOSE REQUIRED FOR MEALS/SNACKS UNDER __G OF CARBS OR EQUAL TO __.__ OR LESS	TIME __ : __ AM / PM LEFT ARM (CGM) / RIGHT ARM (CGM) / LEFT LEG (CGM) / RIGHT LEG (CGM) / LEFT/RIGHT STOMACH (CGM) KETONES NEGATIVE / TRACE / SMALL / MODERATE / LARGE
LUNCH	Total Carbohydrates : ___._ grams	Correction Dose: (BS - ___) / __ (___-___)/__ = (__/__) = ___.__ Carb Dose Calculation: (Meal Carbs / ___) (__._ /___) = ___.__ Correction Dose + Carb Dose Calculation: (___.__ + ___.__) = __.__ OR __ UNITS Correction Dose / Dose Calculation / Rounded to nearest whole number	TIME __ : __ AM / PM LEFT ARM (CGM) / RIGHT ARM (CGM) / LEFT LEG (CGM) / RIGHT LEG (CGM) / LEFT/RIGHT STOMACH (CGM) KETONES NEGATIVE / TRACE / SMALL / MODERATE / LARGE
SNACK	Total Carbohydrates : ___._ grams	Carb Dose Calculation: (Meal Carbs / ___) (__._ /___) = ___.__ or __ UNITS NO INSULIN DOSE REQUIRED FOR MEALS/SNACKS UNDER __G OF CARBS OR EQUAL TO __.__ OR LESS	TIME __ : __ AM / PM LEFT ARM (CGM) / RIGHT ARM (CGM) / LEFT LEG (CGM) / RIGHT LEG (CGM) / LEFT/RIGHT STOMACH (CGM) KETONES NEGATIVE / TRACE / SMALL / MODERATE / LARGE
DINNER	Total Carbohydrates : ___._ grams	Correction Dose: (BS - ___) / __ (___-___)/__ = (__/__) = ___.__ Carb Dose Calculation: (Meal Carbs / ___) (__._ /___) = ___.__ Correction Dose + Carb Dose Calculation: (___.__ + ___.__) = __.__ OR __ UNITS Correction Dose / Dose Calculation / Rounded to nearest whole number	TIME __ : __ AM / PM LEFT ARM (CGM) / RIGHT ARM (CGM) / LEFT LEG (CGM) / RIGHT LEG (CGM) / LEFT/RIGHT STOMACH (CGM) KETONES NEGATIVE / TRACE / SMALL / MODERATE / LARGE
SNACK	Total Carbohydrates : ___._ grams	Carb Dose Calculation: (Meal Carbs / ___) (__._ /___) = ___.__ or __ UNITS NO INSULIN DOSE REQUIRED FOR MEALS/SNACKS UNDER __G OF CARBS OR EQUAL TO __.__ OR LESS	TIME __ : __ AM / PM LEFT ARM (CGM) / RIGHT ARM (CGM) / LEFT LEG (CGM) / RIGHT LEG (CGM) / LEFT/RIGHT STOMACH (CGM) KETONES NEGATIVE / TRACE / SMALL / MODERATE / LARGE
BEDTIME __:__ PM	BLOOD SUGAR ____ UNITS ___ LEFT ARM (CGM) / RIGHT ARM (CGM) / LEFT LEG (CGM) / RIGHT LEG (CGM) / LEFT/RIGHT STOMACH (CGM) KETONES NEGATIVE / TRACE / SMALL / MODERATE / LARGE	HYDRATE 2AM BLOOD SUGAR ____ ADDITIONAL BLOOD SUGAR READINGS BS ___ at __ : __ AM/PM BS ___ at __ : __ AM/PM	NOTES MEDICINE

DATE: ______________________ SUN MON TUES WED THUR FRI SAT

	MEALS AND SNACKS	CARB AND FOOD CALCULATIONS	SHOT DETAILS AND LOCATION
BREAKFAST	Total Carbohydrates : ___._ grams	Correction Dose: (BS - ___) / __ (___-___)/__ = (__/__) = ___.__ Carb Dose Calculation: (Meal Carbs / ___) (__._ /___) = ___.__ Correction Dose + Carb Dose Calculation: (__.__ + __.__) = __.__ OR __ UNITS Correction Dose / Dose Calculation / Rounded to nearest whole number	TIME __ : __ AM / PM LEFT ARM CGM / RIGHT ARM CGM / LEFT LEG CGM / RIGHT LEG CGM / LEFT/RIGHT STOMACH CGM KETONES NEGATIVE / TRACE / SMALL / MODERATE / LARGE
SNACK	Total Carbohydrates : ___._ grams	Carb Dose Calculation: (Meal Carbs / ___) (__._ /___) = ___.__ or __ UNITS NO INSULIN DOSE REQUIRED FOR MEALS/SNACKS UNDER __G OF CARBS OR EQUAL TO __.__ OR LESS	TIME __ : __ AM / PM LEFT ARM CGM / RIGHT ARM CGM / LEFT LEG CGM / RIGHT LEG CGM / LEFT/RIGHT STOMACH CGM KETONES NEGATIVE / TRACE / SMALL / MODERATE / LARGE
LUNCH	Total Carbohydrates : ___._ grams	Correction Dose: (BS - ___) / __ (___-___)/__ = (__/__) = ___.__ Carb Dose Calculation: (Meal Carbs / ___) (__._ /___) = ___.__ Correction Dose + Carb Dose Calculation: (__.__ + __.__) = __.__ OR __ UNITS Correction Dose / Dose Calculation / Rounded to nearest whole number	TIME __ : __ AM / PM LEFT ARM CGM / RIGHT ARM CGM / LEFT LEG CGM / RIGHT LEG CGM / LEFT/RIGHT STOMACH CGM KETONES NEGATIVE / TRACE / SMALL / MODERATE / LARGE
SNACK	Total Carbohydrates : ___._ grams	Carb Dose Calculation: (Meal Carbs / ___) (__._ /___) = ___.__ or __ UNITS NO INSULIN DOSE REQUIRED FOR MEALS/SNACKS UNDER __G OF CARBS OR EQUAL TO __.__ OR LESS	TIME __ : __ AM / PM LEFT ARM CGM / RIGHT ARM CGM / LEFT LEG CGM / RIGHT LEG CGM / LEFT/RIGHT STOMACH CGM KETONES NEGATIVE / TRACE / SMALL / MODERATE / LARGE
DINNER	Total Carbohydrates : ___._ grams	Correction Dose: (BS - ___) / __ (___-___)/__ = (__/__) = ___.__ Carb Dose Calculation: (Meal Carbs / ___) (__._ /___) = ___.__ Correction Dose + Carb Dose Calculation: (__.__ + __.__) = __.__ OR __ UNITS Correction Dose / Dose Calculation / Rounded to nearest whole number	TIME __ : __ AM / PM LEFT ARM CGM / RIGHT ARM CGM / LEFT LEG CGM / RIGHT LEG CGM / LEFT/RIGHT STOMACH CGM KETONES NEGATIVE / TRACE / SMALL / MODERATE / LARGE
SNACK	Total Carbohydrates : ___._ grams	Carb Dose Calculation: (Meal Carbs / ___) (__._ /___) = ___.__ or __ UNITS NO INSULIN DOSE REQUIRED FOR MEALS/SNACKS UNDER __G OF CARBS OR EQUAL TO __.__ OR LESS	TIME __ : __ AM / PM LEFT ARM CGM / RIGHT ARM CGM / LEFT LEG CGM / RIGHT LEG CGM / LEFT/RIGHT STOMACH CGM KETONES NEGATIVE / TRACE / SMALL / MODERATE / LARGE
BEDTIME __ : __ PM	BLOOD SUGAR _____ UNITS ___ LEFT ARM CGM / RIGHT ARM CGM / LEFT LEG CGM / RIGHT LEG CGM / LEFT/RIGHT STOMACH CGM KETONES NEGATIVE / TRACE / SMALL / MODERATE / LARGE	HYDRATE 2AM BLOOD SUGAR _____ ADDITIONAL BLOOD SUGAR READINGS BS ___ at __ : __ AM/PM BS ___ at __ : __ AM/PM	NOTES MEDICINE

DATE: ______________________ SUN MON TUES WED THUR FRI SAT

	MEALS AND SNACKS	CARB AND FOOD CALCULATIONS	SHOT DETAILS AND LOCATION
BREAKFAST	Total Carbohydrates : ___._ grams	Correction Dose: (BS - ___) / __ (___-___)/__ = (__/__) = ___.__ Carb Dose Calculation: (Meal Carbs / ___) (__._ /___) = ___.__ Correction Dose + Carb Dose Calculation: (_____ + _____) = __.__ OR __ UNITS Correction Dose · Dose Calculation · Rounded to nearest whole number	TIME __ : __ AM / PM LEFT ARM CGM · RIGHT ARM CGM · LEFT LEG CGM · RIGHT LEG CGM · LEFT/RIGHT STOMACH CGM KETONES NEGATIVE · TRACE · SMALL · MODERATE · LARGE
SNACK	Total Carbohydrates : ___._ grams	Carb Dose Calculation: (Meal Carbs / ___) (__._ /___) = ___.__ or __ UNITS NO INSULIN DOSE REQUIRED FOR MEALS/SNACKS UNDER __G OF CARBS OR EQUAL TO __.__ OR LESS	TIME __ : __ AM / PM LEFT ARM CGM · RIGHT ARM CGM · LEFT LEG CGM · RIGHT LEG CGM · LEFT/RIGHT STOMACH CGM KETONES NEGATIVE · TRACE · SMALL · MODERATE · LARGE
LUNCH	Total Carbohydrates : ___._ grams	Correction Dose: (BS - ___) / __ (___-___)/__ = (__/__) = ___.__ Carb Dose Calculation: (Meal Carbs / ___) (__._ /___) = ___.__ Correction Dose + Carb Dose Calculation: (_____ + _____) = __.__ OR __ UNITS Correction Dose · Dose Calculation · Rounded to nearest whole number	TIME __ : __ AM / PM LEFT ARM CGM · RIGHT ARM CGM · LEFT LEG CGM · RIGHT LEG CGM · LEFT/RIGHT STOMACH CGM KETONES NEGATIVE · TRACE · SMALL · MODERATE · LARGE
SNACK	Total Carbohydrates : ___._ grams	Carb Dose Calculation: (Meal Carbs / ___) (__._ /___) = ___.__ or __ UNITS NO INSULIN DOSE REQUIRED FOR MEALS/SNACKS UNDER __G OF CARBS OR EQUAL TO __.__ OR LESS	TIME __ : __ AM / PM LEFT ARM CGM · RIGHT ARM CGM · LEFT LEG CGM · RIGHT LEG CGM · LEFT/RIGHT STOMACH CGM KETONES NEGATIVE · TRACE · SMALL · MODERATE · LARGE
DINNER	Total Carbohydrates : ___._ grams	Correction Dose: (BS - ___) / __ (___-___)/__ = (__/__) = ___.__ Carb Dose Calculation: (Meal Carbs / ___) (__._ /___) = ___.__ Correction Dose + Carb Dose Calculation: (_____ + _____) = __.__ OR __ UNITS Correction Dose · Dose Calculation · Rounded to nearest whole number	TIME __ : __ AM / PM LEFT ARM CGM · RIGHT ARM CGM · LEFT LEG CGM · RIGHT LEG CGM · LEFT/RIGHT STOMACH CGM KETONES NEGATIVE · TRACE · SMALL · MODERATE · LARGE
SNACK	Total Carbohydrates : ___._ grams	Carb Dose Calculation: (Meal Carbs / ___) (__._ /___) = ___.__ or __ UNITS NO INSULIN DOSE REQUIRED FOR MEALS/SNACKS UNDER __G OF CARBS OR EQUAL TO __.__ OR LESS	TIME __ : __ AM / PM LEFT ARM CGM · RIGHT ARM CGM · LEFT LEG CGM · RIGHT LEG CGM · LEFT/RIGHT STOMACH CGM KETONES NEGATIVE · TRACE · SMALL · MODERATE · LARGE
BEDTIME __ : __ PM	BLOOD SUGAR _____ UNITS ___ LEFT ARM CGM · RIGHT ARM CGM · LEFT LEG CGM · RIGHT LEG CGM · LEFT/RIGHT STOMACH CGM KETONES NEGATIVE · TRACE · SMALL · MODERATE · LARGE	HYDRATE 2AM BLOOD SUGAR _____ ADDITIONAL BLOOD SUGAR READINGS BS ___ at __ : __ AM/PM BS ___ at __ : __ AM/PM	NOTES MEDICINE

DATE: ______________________ SUN MON TUES WED THUR FRI SAT

	MEALS AND SNACKS	CARB AND FOOD CALCULATIONS	SHOT DETAILS AND LOCATION
BREAKFAST	Total Carbohydrates : ___._ grams	Correction Dose: (BS - ___) / __ (___-___)/__ = (__/__) = ___.__ Carb Dose Calculation: (Meal Carbs / ___) (__._ /___) = ___.__ Correction Dose + Carb Dose Calculation: (_____ + _____) = __.__ OR __ UNITS Correction Dose / Dose Calculation / Rounded to nearest whole number	TIME __ : __ AM / PM LEFT ARM CGM / RIGHT ARM CGM / LEFT LEG CGM / RIGHT LEG CGM / LEFT/RIGHT STOMACH CGM KETONES NEGATIVE / TRACE / SMALL / MODERATE / LARGE
SNACK	Total Carbohydrates : ___._ grams	Carb Dose Calculation: (Meal Carbs / ___) (__._ /___) = ___.__ or __ UNITS NO INSULIN DOSE REQUIRED FOR MEALS/SNACKS UNDER __G OF CARBS OR EQUAL TO __.__ OR LESS	TIME __ : __ AM / PM LEFT ARM CGM / RIGHT ARM CGM / LEFT LEG CGM / RIGHT LEG CGM / LEFT/RIGHT STOMACH CGM KETONES NEGATIVE / TRACE / SMALL / MODERATE / LARGE
LUNCH	Total Carbohydrates : ___._ grams	Correction Dose: (BS - ___) / __ (___-___)/__ = (__/__) = ___.__ Carb Dose Calculation: (Meal Carbs / ___) (__._ /___) = ___.__ Correction Dose + Carb Dose Calculation: (_____ + _____) = __.__ OR __ UNITS Correction Dose / Dose Calculation / Rounded to nearest whole number	TIME __ : __ AM / PM LEFT ARM CGM / RIGHT ARM CGM / LEFT LEG CGM / RIGHT LEG CGM / LEFT/RIGHT STOMACH CGM KETONES NEGATIVE / TRACE / SMALL / MODERATE / LARGE
SNACK	Total Carbohydrates : ___._ grams	Carb Dose Calculation: (Meal Carbs / ___) (__._ /___) = ___.__ or __ UNITS NO INSULIN DOSE REQUIRED FOR MEALS/SNACKS UNDER __G OF CARBS OR EQUAL TO __.__ OR LESS	TIME __ : __ AM / PM LEFT ARM CGM / RIGHT ARM CGM / LEFT LEG CGM / RIGHT LEG CGM / LEFT/RIGHT STOMACH CGM KETONES NEGATIVE / TRACE / SMALL / MODERATE / LARGE
DINNER	Total Carbohydrates : ___._ grams	Correction Dose: (BS - ___) / __ (___-___)/__ = (__/__) = ___.__ Carb Dose Calculation: (Meal Carbs / ___) (__._ /___) = ___.__ Correction Dose + Carb Dose Calculation: (_____ + _____) = __.__ OR __ UNITS Correction Dose / Dose Calculation / Rounded to nearest whole number	TIME __ : __ AM / PM LEFT ARM CGM / RIGHT ARM CGM / LEFT LEG CGM / RIGHT LEG CGM / LEFT/RIGHT STOMACH CGM KETONES NEGATIVE / TRACE / SMALL / MODERATE / LARGE
SNACK	Total Carbohydrates : ___._ grams	Carb Dose Calculation: (Meal Carbs / ___) (__._ /___) = ___.__ or __ UNITS NO INSULIN DOSE REQUIRED FOR MEALS/SNACKS UNDER __G OF CARBS OR EQUAL TO __.__ OR LESS	TIME __ : __ AM / PM LEFT ARM CGM / RIGHT ARM CGM / LEFT LEG CGM / RIGHT LEG CGM / LEFT/RIGHT STOMACH CGM KETONES NEGATIVE / TRACE / SMALL / MODERATE / LARGE
BEDTIME __ : __ PM	BLOOD SUGAR _____ UNITS ___ LEFT ARM CGM / RIGHT ARM CGM / LEFT LEG CGM / RIGHT LEG CGM / LEFT/RIGHT STOMACH CGM KETONES NEGATIVE / TRACE / SMALL / MODERATE / LARGE	HYDRATE 2AM BLOOD SUGAR _____ ADDITIONAL BLOOD SUGAR READINGS BS ___ at __ : __ AM/PM BS ___ at __ : __ AM/PM	NOTES MEDICINE

DATE: ______________________ SUN MON TUES WED THUR FRI SAT

	MEALS AND SNACKS	CARB AND FOOD CALCULATIONS	SHOT DETAILS AND LOCATION
BREAKFAST	Total Carbohydrates : ___._ grams	Correction Dose: (BS - ___) / __ (___-___)/__ = (__/__) = ___.__ Carb Dose Calculation: (Meal Carbs / ___) (__._ /___) = ___.__ Correction Dose + Carb Dose Calculation: (__.__ + __.__) = __.__ OR __ UNITS Correction Dose / Dose Calculation / Rounded to nearest whole number	TIME __ : __ AM / PM LEFT ARM CGM / RIGHT ARM CGM / LEFT LEG CGM / RIGHT LEG CGM / LEFT/RIGHT STOMACH CGM KETONES NEGATIVE / TRACE / SMALL / MODERATE / LARGE
SNACK	Total Carbohydrates : ___._ grams	Carb Dose Calculation: (Meal Carbs / ___) (__._ /___) = ___.__ or __ UNITS NO INSULIN DOSE REQUIRED FOR MEALS/SNACKS UNDER __G OF CARBS OR EQUAL TO __.__ OR LESS	TIME __ : __ AM / PM LEFT ARM CGM / RIGHT ARM CGM / LEFT LEG CGM / RIGHT LEG CGM / LEFT/RIGHT STOMACH CGM KETONES NEGATIVE / TRACE / SMALL / MODERATE / LARGE
LUNCH	Total Carbohydrates : ___._ grams	Correction Dose: (BS - ___) / __ (___-___)/__ = (__/__) = ___.__ Carb Dose Calculation: (Meal Carbs / ___) (__._ /___) = ___.__ Correction Dose + Carb Dose Calculation: (__.__ + __.__) = __.__ OR __ UNITS Correction Dose / Dose Calculation / Rounded to nearest whole number	TIME __ : __ AM / PM LEFT ARM CGM / RIGHT ARM CGM / LEFT LEG CGM / RIGHT LEG CGM / LEFT/RIGHT STOMACH CGM KETONES NEGATIVE / TRACE / SMALL / MODERATE / LARGE
SNACK	Total Carbohydrates : ___._ grams	Carb Dose Calculation: (Meal Carbs / ___) (__._ /___) = ___.__ or __ UNITS NO INSULIN DOSE REQUIRED FOR MEALS/SNACKS UNDER __G OF CARBS OR EQUAL TO __.__ OR LESS	TIME __ : __ AM / PM LEFT ARM CGM / RIGHT ARM CGM / LEFT LEG CGM / RIGHT LEG CGM / LEFT/RIGHT STOMACH CGM KETONES NEGATIVE / TRACE / SMALL / MODERATE / LARGE
DINNER	Total Carbohydrates : ___._ grams	Correction Dose: (BS - ___) / __ (___-___)/__ = (__/__) = ___.__ Carb Dose Calculation: (Meal Carbs / ___) (__._ /___) = ___.__ Correction Dose + Carb Dose Calculation: (__.__ + __.__) = __.__ OR __ UNITS Correction Dose / Dose Calculation / Rounded to nearest whole number	TIME __ : __ AM / PM LEFT ARM CGM / RIGHT ARM CGM / LEFT LEG CGM / RIGHT LEG CGM / LEFT/RIGHT STOMACH CGM KETONES NEGATIVE / TRACE / SMALL / MODERATE / LARGE
SNACK	Total Carbohydrates : ___._ grams	Carb Dose Calculation: (Meal Carbs / ___) (__._ /___) = ___.__ or __ UNITS NO INSULIN DOSE REQUIRED FOR MEALS/SNACKS UNDER __G OF CARBS OR EQUAL TO __.__ OR LESS	TIME __ : __ AM / PM LEFT ARM CGM / RIGHT ARM CGM / LEFT LEG CGM / RIGHT LEG CGM / LEFT/RIGHT STOMACH CGM KETONES NEGATIVE / TRACE / SMALL / MODERATE / LARGE
BEDTIME __ : __ PM	BLOOD SUGAR _____ UNITS ___ LEFT ARM CGM / RIGHT ARM CGM / LEFT LEG CGM / RIGHT LEG CGM / LEFT/RIGHT STOMACH CGM KETONES NEGATIVE / TRACE / SMALL / MODERATE / LARGE	HYDRATE 2AM BLOOD SUGAR _____ ADDITIONAL BLOOD SUGAR READINGS BS ___ at __ : __ AM/PM BS ___ at __ : __ AM/PM	NOTES MEDICINE

DATE: ______________________ SUN MON TUES WED THUR FRI SAT

	MEALS AND SNACKS	CARB AND FOOD CALCULATIONS	SHOT DETAILS AND LOCATION
BREAKFAST	Total Carbohydrates : ___._ grams	Correction Dose: (BS - ___) / __ (___-___)/__ = (__/__) = ___.__ Carb Dose Calculation: (Meal Carbs / ___) (__._ /___) = ___.__ Correction Dose + Carb Dose Calculation: (___.__ + _____) = __.__ OR __ UNITS Correction Dose / Dose Calculation / Rounded to nearest whole number	TIME __ : __ AM / PM LEFT ARM CGM / RIGHT ARM CGM / LEFT LEG CGM / RIGHT LEG CGM / LEFT/RIGHT STOMACH CGM KETONES NEGATIVE / TRACE / SMALL / MODERATE / LARGE
SNACK	Total Carbohydrates : ___._ grams	Carb Dose Calculation: (Meal Carbs / ___) (__._ /___) = ___.__ or __ UNITS NO INSULIN DOSE REQUIRED FOR MEALS/SNACKS UNDER __G OF CARBS OR EQUAL TO __.__ OR LESS	TIME __ : __ AM / PM LEFT ARM CGM / RIGHT ARM CGM / LEFT LEG CGM / RIGHT LEG CGM / LEFT/RIGHT STOMACH CGM KETONES NEGATIVE / TRACE / SMALL / MODERATE / LARGE
LUNCH	Total Carbohydrates : ___._ grams	Correction Dose: (BS - ___) / __ (___-___)/__ = (__/__) = ___.__ Carb Dose Calculation: (Meal Carbs / ___) (__._ /___) = ___.__ Correction Dose + Carb Dose Calculation: (___.__ + _____) = __.__ OR __ UNITS Correction Dose / Dose Calculation / Rounded to nearest whole number	TIME __ : __ AM / PM LEFT ARM CGM / RIGHT ARM CGM / LEFT LEG CGM / RIGHT LEG CGM / LEFT/RIGHT STOMACH CGM KETONES NEGATIVE / TRACE / SMALL / MODERATE / LARGE
SNACK	Total Carbohydrates : ___._ grams	Carb Dose Calculation: (Meal Carbs / ___) (__._ /___) = ___.__ or __ UNITS NO INSULIN DOSE REQUIRED FOR MEALS/SNACKS UNDER __G OF CARBS OR EQUAL TO __.__ OR LESS	TIME __ : __ AM / PM LEFT ARM CGM / RIGHT ARM CGM / LEFT LEG CGM / RIGHT LEG CGM / LEFT/RIGHT STOMACH CGM KETONES NEGATIVE / TRACE / SMALL / MODERATE / LARGE
DINNER	Total Carbohydrates : ___._ grams	Correction Dose: (BS - ___) / __ (___-___)/__ = (__/__) = ___.__ Carb Dose Calculation: (Meal Carbs / ___) (__._ /___) = ___.__ Correction Dose + Carb Dose Calculation: (___.__ + _____) = __.__ OR __ UNITS Correction Dose / Dose Calculation / Rounded to nearest whole number	TIME __ : __ AM / PM LEFT ARM CGM / RIGHT ARM CGM / LEFT LEG CGM / RIGHT LEG CGM / LEFT/RIGHT STOMACH CGM KETONES NEGATIVE / TRACE / SMALL / MODERATE / LARGE
SNACK	Total Carbohydrates : ___._ grams	Carb Dose Calculation: (Meal Carbs / ___) (__._ /___) = ___.__ or __ UNITS NO INSULIN DOSE REQUIRED FOR MEALS/SNACKS UNDER __G OF CARBS OR EQUAL TO __.__ OR LESS	TIME __ : __ AM / PM LEFT ARM CGM / RIGHT ARM CGM / LEFT LEG CGM / RIGHT LEG CGM / LEFT/RIGHT STOMACH CGM KETONES NEGATIVE / TRACE / SMALL / MODERATE / LARGE
BEDTIME __ : __ PM	BLOOD SUGAR _____ UNITS ___ LEFT ARM CGM / RIGHT ARM CGM / LEFT LEG CGM / RIGHT LEG CGM / LEFT/RIGHT STOMACH CGM KETONES NEGATIVE / TRACE / SMALL / MODERATE / LARGE	HYDRATE 2AM BLOOD SUGAR _____ ADDITIONAL BLOOD SUGAR READINGS BS ___ at __ : __ AM/PM BS ___ at __ : __ AM/PM	NOTES MEDICINE

DATE: ____________________ SUN MON TUES WED THUR FRI SAT

	MEALS AND SNACKS	CARB AND FOOD CALCULATIONS	SHOT DETAILS AND LOCATION
BREAKFAST	Total Carbohydrates : ___._ grams	Correction Dose: (BS - ___) / __ (___-___)/__ = (__/__) = ___.__ Carb Dose Calculation: (Meal Carbs / ___) (__._ /___) = ___.__ Correction Dose + Carb Dose Calculation: (______ + ______) = __.__ OR __ UNITS Correction Dose / Dose Calculation / Rounded to nearest whole number	TIME __:__ AM / PM LEFT ARM CGM / RIGHT ARM CGM / LEFT LEG CGM / RIGHT LEG CGM / LEFT/RIGHT STOMACH CGM KETONES NEGATIVE TRACE SMALL MODERATE LARGE
SNACK	Total Carbohydrates : ___._ grams	Carb Dose Calculation: (Meal Carbs / ___) (__._ /___) = ___.__ or __ UNITS NO INSULIN DOSE REQUIRED FOR MEALS/SNACKS UNDER __G OF CARBS OR EQUAL TO __.__ OR LESS	TIME __:__ AM / PM LEFT ARM CGM / RIGHT ARM CGM / LEFT LEG CGM / RIGHT LEG CGM / LEFT/RIGHT STOMACH CGM KETONES NEGATIVE TRACE SMALL MODERATE LARGE
LUNCH	Total Carbohydrates : ___._ grams	Correction Dose: (BS - ___) / __ (___-___)/__ = (__/__) = ___.__ Carb Dose Calculation: (Meal Carbs / ___) (__._ /___) = ___.__ Correction Dose + Carb Dose Calculation: (______ + ______) = __.__ OR __ UNITS Correction Dose / Dose Calculation / Rounded to nearest whole number	TIME __:__ AM / PM LEFT ARM CGM / RIGHT ARM CGM / LEFT LEG CGM / RIGHT LEG CGM / LEFT/RIGHT STOMACH CGM KETONES NEGATIVE TRACE SMALL MODERATE LARGE
SNACK	Total Carbohydrates : ___._ grams	Carb Dose Calculation: (Meal Carbs / ___) (__._ /___) = ___.__ or __ UNITS NO INSULIN DOSE REQUIRED FOR MEALS/SNACKS UNDER __G OF CARBS OR EQUAL TO __.__ OR LESS	TIME __:__ AM / PM LEFT ARM CGM / RIGHT ARM CGM / LEFT LEG CGM / RIGHT LEG CGM / LEFT/RIGHT STOMACH CGM KETONES NEGATIVE TRACE SMALL MODERATE LARGE
DINNER	Total Carbohydrates : ___._ grams	Correction Dose: (BS - ___) / __ (___-___)/__ = (__/__) = ___.__ Carb Dose Calculation: (Meal Carbs / ___) (__._ /___) = ___.__ Correction Dose + Carb Dose Calculation: (______ + ______) = __.__ OR __ UNITS Correction Dose / Dose Calculation / Rounded to nearest whole number	TIME __:__ AM / PM LEFT ARM CGM / RIGHT ARM CGM / LEFT LEG CGM / RIGHT LEG CGM / LEFT/RIGHT STOMACH CGM KETONES NEGATIVE TRACE SMALL MODERATE LARGE
SNACK	Total Carbohydrates : ___._ grams	Carb Dose Calculation: (Meal Carbs / ___) (__._ /___) = ___.__ or __ UNITS NO INSULIN DOSE REQUIRED FOR MEALS/SNACKS UNDER __G OF CARBS OR EQUAL TO __.__ OR LESS	TIME __:__ AM / PM LEFT ARM CGM / RIGHT ARM CGM / LEFT LEG CGM / RIGHT LEG CGM / LEFT/RIGHT STOMACH CGM KETONES NEGATIVE TRACE SMALL MODERATE LARGE
BEDTIME __:__ PM	BLOOD SUGAR ____ UNITS __ LEFT ARM CGM / RIGHT ARM CGM / LEFT LEG CGM / RIGHT LEG CGM / LEFT/RIGHT STOMACH CGM KETONES NEGATIVE TRACE SMALL MODERATE LARGE	HYDRATE 2AM BLOOD SUGAR ____ ADDITIONAL BLOOD SUGAR READINGS BS ___ at __ : __ AM/PM BS ___ at __ : __ AM/PM	NOTES MEDICINE

DATE: ______________________ SUN MON TUES WED THUR FRI SAT

	MEALS AND SNACKS	CARB AND FOOD CALCULATIONS	SHOT DETAILS AND LOCATION
BREAKFAST	Total Carbohydrates : ___._ grams	Correction Dose: (BS - ___) / __ (___-___)/__ = (__/__) = ___.__ Carb Dose Calculation: (Meal Carbs / ___) (__._ /___) = ___.__ Correction Dose + Carb Dose Calculation: (_____ + _____) = __.__ OR __ UNITS Correction Dose / Dose Calculation / Rounded to nearest whole number	TIME __ : __ AM / PM LEFT ARM CGM / RIGHT ARM CGM / LEFT LEG CGM / RIGHT LEG CGM / LEFT/RIGHT STOMACH CGM KETONES NEGATIVE TRACE SMALL MODERATE LARGE
SNACK	Total Carbohydrates : ___._ grams	Carb Dose Calculation: (Meal Carbs / ___) (__._ /___) = ___.__ or __ UNITS NO INSULIN DOSE REQUIRED FOR MEALS/SNACKS UNDER __G OF CARBS OR EQUAL TO __.__ OR LESS	TIME __ : __ AM / PM LEFT ARM CGM / RIGHT ARM CGM / LEFT LEG CGM / RIGHT LEG CGM / LEFT/RIGHT STOMACH CGM KETONES NEGATIVE TRACE SMALL MODERATE LARGE
LUNCH	Total Carbohydrates : ___._ grams	Correction Dose: (BS - ___) / __ (___-___)/__ = (__/__) = ___.__ Carb Dose Calculation: (Meal Carbs / ___) (__._ /___) = ___.__ Correction Dose + Carb Dose Calculation: (_____ + _____) = __.__ OR __ UNITS Correction Dose / Dose Calculation / Rounded to nearest whole number	TIME __ : __ AM / PM LEFT ARM CGM / RIGHT ARM CGM / LEFT LEG CGM / RIGHT LEG CGM / LEFT/RIGHT STOMACH CGM KETONES NEGATIVE TRACE SMALL MODERATE LARGE
SNACK	Total Carbohydrates : ___._ grams	Carb Dose Calculation: (Meal Carbs / ___) (__._ /___) = ___.__ or __ UNITS NO INSULIN DOSE REQUIRED FOR MEALS/SNACKS UNDER __G OF CARBS OR EQUAL TO __.__ OR LESS	TIME __ : __ AM / PM LEFT ARM CGM / RIGHT ARM CGM / LEFT LEG CGM / RIGHT LEG CGM / LEFT/RIGHT STOMACH CGM KETONES NEGATIVE TRACE SMALL MODERATE LARGE
DINNER	Total Carbohydrates : ___._ grams	Correction Dose: (BS - ___) / __ (___-___)/__ = (__/__) = ___.__ Carb Dose Calculation: (Meal Carbs / ___) (__._ /___) = ___.__ Correction Dose + Carb Dose Calculation: (_____ + _____) = __.__ OR __ UNITS Correction Dose / Dose Calculation / Rounded to nearest whole number	TIME __ : __ AM / PM LEFT ARM CGM / RIGHT ARM CGM / LEFT LEG CGM / RIGHT LEG CGM / LEFT/RIGHT STOMACH CGM KETONES NEGATIVE TRACE SMALL MODERATE LARGE
SNACK	Total Carbohydrates : ___._ grams	Carb Dose Calculation: (Meal Carbs / ___) (__._ /___) = ___.__ or __ UNITS NO INSULIN DOSE REQUIRED FOR MEALS/SNACKS UNDER __G OF CARBS OR EQUAL TO __.__ OR LESS	TIME __ : __ AM / PM LEFT ARM CGM / RIGHT ARM CGM / LEFT LEG CGM / RIGHT LEG CGM / LEFT/RIGHT STOMACH CGM KETONES NEGATIVE TRACE SMALL MODERATE LARGE
BEDTIME __ : __ PM	BLOOD SUGAR ______ UNITS ___ LEFT ARM CGM / RIGHT ARM CGM / LEFT LEG CGM / RIGHT LEG CGM / LEFT/RIGHT STOMACH CGM KETONES NEGATIVE TRACE SMALL MODERATE LARGE	HYDRATE 2AM BLOOD SUGAR _____ ADDITIONAL BLOOD SUGAR READINGS BS ___ at __ : __ AM/PM BS ___ at __ : __ AM/PM	NOTES MEDICINE

DATE: ______________________ SUN MON TUES WED THUR FRI SAT

	MEALS AND SNACKS	CARB AND FOOD CALCULATIONS	SHOT DETAILS AND LOCATION
BREAKFAST	Total Carbohydrates : ___._ grams	Correction Dose: (BS - ___) / __ (___-___)/__ = (__/__) = ___.__ Carb Dose Calculation: (Meal Carbs / ___) (__._ /___) = ___.__ Correction Dose + Carb Dose Calculation: (_____ + _____) = __.__ OR __ UNITS Correction Dose / Dose Calculation / Rounded to nearest whole number	TIME __ :__ AM / PM LEFT ARM CGM / RIGHT ARM CGM / LEFT LEG CGM / RIGHT LEG CGM / LEFT/RIGHT STOMACH CGM KETONES NEGATIVE / TRACE / SMALL / MODERATE / LARGE
SNACK	Total Carbohydrates : ___._ grams	Carb Dose Calculation: (Meal Carbs / ___) (__._ /___) = ___.__ or __ UNITS NO INSULIN DOSE REQUIRED FOR MEALS/SNACKS UNDER __G OF CARBS OR EQUAL TO __.__ OR LESS	TIME __ :__ AM / PM LEFT ARM CGM / RIGHT ARM CGM / LEFT LEG CGM / RIGHT LEG CGM / LEFT/RIGHT STOMACH CGM KETONES NEGATIVE / TRACE / SMALL / MODERATE / LARGE
LUNCH	Total Carbohydrates : ___._ grams	Correction Dose: (BS - ___) / __ (___-___)/__ = (__/__) = ___.__ Carb Dose Calculation: (Meal Carbs / ___) (__._ /___) = ___.__ Correction Dose + Carb Dose Calculation: (_____ + _____) = __.__ OR __ UNITS Correction Dose / Dose Calculation / Rounded to nearest whole number	TIME __ :__ AM / PM LEFT ARM CGM / RIGHT ARM CGM / LEFT LEG CGM / RIGHT LEG CGM / LEFT/RIGHT STOMACH CGM KETONES NEGATIVE / TRACE / SMALL / MODERATE / LARGE
SNACK	Total Carbohydrates : ___._ grams	Carb Dose Calculation: (Meal Carbs / ___) (__._ /___) = ___.__ or __ UNITS NO INSULIN DOSE REQUIRED FOR MEALS/SNACKS UNDER __G OF CARBS OR EQUAL TO __.__ OR LESS	TIME __ :__ AM / PM LEFT ARM CGM / RIGHT ARM CGM / LEFT LEG CGM / RIGHT LEG CGM / LEFT/RIGHT STOMACH CGM KETONES NEGATIVE / TRACE / SMALL / MODERATE / LARGE
DINNER	Total Carbohydrates : ___._ grams	Correction Dose: (BS - ___) / __ (___-___)/__ = (__/__) = ___.__ Carb Dose Calculation: (Meal Carbs / ___) (__._ /___) = ___.__ Correction Dose + Carb Dose Calculation: (_____ + _____) = __.__ OR __ UNITS Correction Dose / Dose Calculation / Rounded to nearest whole number	TIME __ :__ AM / PM LEFT ARM CGM / RIGHT ARM CGM / LEFT LEG CGM / RIGHT LEG CGM / LEFT/RIGHT STOMACH CGM KETONES NEGATIVE / TRACE / SMALL / MODERATE / LARGE
SNACK	Total Carbohydrates : ___._ grams	Carb Dose Calculation: (Meal Carbs / ___) (__._ /___) = ___.__ or __ UNITS NO INSULIN DOSE REQUIRED FOR MEALS/SNACKS UNDER __G OF CARBS OR EQUAL TO __.__ OR LESS	TIME __ :__ AM / PM LEFT ARM CGM / RIGHT ARM CGM / LEFT LEG CGM / RIGHT LEG CGM / LEFT/RIGHT STOMACH CGM KETONES NEGATIVE / TRACE / SMALL / MODERATE / LARGE
BEDTIME __ : __ PM	BLOOD SUGAR ____ UNITS __ LEFT ARM CGM / RIGHT ARM CGM / LEFT LEG CGM / RIGHT LEG CGM / LEFT/RIGHT STOMACH CGM KETONES NEGATIVE / TRACE / SMALL / MODERATE / LARGE	HYDRATE 2AM BLOOD SUGAR ____ ADDITIONAL BLOOD SUGAR READINGS BS ___ at __ : __ AM/PM BS ___ at __ : __ AM/PM	NOTES MEDICINE

DATE: ______________________________ SUN MON TUES WED THUR FRI SAT

	MEALS AND SNACKS	CARB AND FOOD CALCULATIONS	SHOT DETAILS AND LOCATION
BREAKFAST	Total Carbohydrates : ___.__ grams	Correction Dose: (BS - ___) / __ (___-___)/__ = (__/__) = ___.__ Carb Dose Calculation: (Meal Carbs / ___) (__.__ /___) = ___.__ Correction Dose + Carb Dose Calculation: (__.__ + __.__) = __.__ OR __ UNITS Correction Dose · Dose Calculation · Rounded to nearest whole number	TIME __ : __ AM / PM LEFT ARM CGM · RIGHT ARM CGM · LEFT LEG CGM · RIGHT LEG CGM · LEFT/RIGHT STOMACH CGM KETONES NEGATIVE · TRACE · SMALL · MODERATE · LARGE
SNACK	Total Carbohydrates : ___.__ grams	Carb Dose Calculation: (Meal Carbs / ___) (__.__ /___) = ___.__ or __ UNITS NO INSULIN DOSE REQUIRED FOR MEALS/SNACKS UNDER __G OF CARBS OR EQUAL TO __.__ OR LESS	TIME __ : __ AM / PM LEFT ARM CGM · RIGHT ARM CGM · LEFT LEG CGM · RIGHT LEG CGM · LEFT/RIGHT STOMACH CGM KETONES NEGATIVE · TRACE · SMALL · MODERATE · LARGE
LUNCH	Total Carbohydrates : ___.__ grams	Correction Dose: (BS - ___) / __ (___-___)/__ = (__/__) = ___.__ Carb Dose Calculation: (Meal Carbs / ___) (__.__ /___) = ___.__ Correction Dose + Carb Dose Calculation: (__.__ + __.__) = __.__ OR __ UNITS Correction Dose · Dose Calculation · Rounded to nearest whole number	TIME __ : __ AM / PM LEFT ARM CGM · RIGHT ARM CGM · LEFT LEG CGM · RIGHT LEG CGM · LEFT/RIGHT STOMACH CGM KETONES NEGATIVE · TRACE · SMALL · MODERATE · LARGE
SNACK	Total Carbohydrates : ___.__ grams	Carb Dose Calculation: (Meal Carbs / ___) (__.__ /___) = ___.__ or __ UNITS NO INSULIN DOSE REQUIRED FOR MEALS/SNACKS UNDER __G OF CARBS OR EQUAL TO __.__ OR LESS	TIME __ : __ AM / PM LEFT ARM CGM · RIGHT ARM CGM · LEFT LEG CGM · RIGHT LEG CGM · LEFT/RIGHT STOMACH CGM KETONES NEGATIVE · TRACE · SMALL · MODERATE · LARGE
DINNER	Total Carbohydrates : ___.__ grams	Correction Dose: (BS - ___) / __ (___-___)/__ = (__/__) = ___.__ Carb Dose Calculation: (Meal Carbs / ___) (__.__ /___) = ___.__ Correction Dose + Carb Dose Calculation: (__.__ + __.__) = __.__ OR __ UNITS Correction Dose · Dose Calculation · Rounded to nearest whole number	TIME __ : __ AM / PM LEFT ARM CGM · RIGHT ARM CGM · LEFT LEG CGM · RIGHT LEG CGM · LEFT/RIGHT STOMACH CGM KETONES NEGATIVE · TRACE · SMALL · MODERATE · LARGE
SNACK	Total Carbohydrates : ___.__ grams	Carb Dose Calculation: (Meal Carbs / ___) (__.__ /___) = ___.__ or __ UNITS NO INSULIN DOSE REQUIRED FOR MEALS/SNACKS UNDER __G OF CARBS OR EQUAL TO __.__ OR LESS	TIME __ : __ AM / PM LEFT ARM CGM · RIGHT ARM CGM · LEFT LEG CGM · RIGHT LEG CGM · LEFT/RIGHT STOMACH CGM KETONES NEGATIVE · TRACE · SMALL · MODERATE · LARGE
BEDTIME __ : __ PM	BLOOD SUGAR _____ UNITS ___ LEFT ARM CGM · RIGHT ARM CGM · LEFT LEG CGM · RIGHT LEG CGM · LEFT/RIGHT STOMACH CGM KETONES NEGATIVE · TRACE · SMALL · MODERATE · LARGE	HYDRATE 2AM BLOOD SUGAR _____ ADDITIONAL BLOOD SUGAR READINGS BS ___ at __ : __ AM/PM BS ___ at __ : __ AM/PM	NOTES MEDICINE

DATE: ______________________ SUN MON TUES WED THUR FRI SAT

	MEALS AND SNACKS	CARB AND FOOD CALCULATIONS	SHOT DETAILS AND LOCATION
BREAKFAST	Total Carbohydrates : ___._ grams	Correction Dose: (BS - ___) / __ (___-___)/__ = (__/__) = ___.__ Carb Dose Calculation: (Meal Carbs / ___) (__._ /___) = ___.__ Correction Dose + Carb Dose Calculation: (_____ + _____) = __.__ OR __ UNITS Correction Dose / Dose Calculation / Rounded to nearest whole number	TIME __:__ AM / PM LEFT ARM CGM / RIGHT ARM CGM / LEFT LEG CGM / RIGHT LEG CGM / LEFT/RIGHT STOMACH CGM KETONES NEGATIVE TRACE SMALL MODERATE LARGE
SNACK	Total Carbohydrates : ___._ grams	Carb Dose Calculation: (Meal Carbs / ___) (__._ /___) = ___.__ or __ UNITS NO INSULIN DOSE REQUIRED FOR MEALS/SNACKS UNDER __G OF CARBS OR EQUAL TO __.__ OR LESS	TIME __:__ AM / PM LEFT ARM CGM / RIGHT ARM CGM / LEFT LEG CGM / RIGHT LEG CGM / LEFT/RIGHT STOMACH CGM KETONES NEGATIVE TRACE SMALL MODERATE LARGE
LUNCH	Total Carbohydrates : ___._ grams	Correction Dose: (BS - ___) / __ (___-___)/__ = (__/__) = ___.__ Carb Dose Calculation: (Meal Carbs / ___) (__._ /___) = ___.__ Correction Dose + Carb Dose Calculation: (_____ + _____) = __.__ OR __ UNITS Correction Dose / Dose Calculation / Rounded to nearest whole number	TIME __:__ AM / PM LEFT ARM CGM / RIGHT ARM CGM / LEFT LEG CGM / RIGHT LEG CGM / LEFT/RIGHT STOMACH CGM KETONES NEGATIVE TRACE SMALL MODERATE LARGE
SNACK	Total Carbohydrates : ___._ grams	Carb Dose Calculation: (Meal Carbs / ___) (__._ /___) = ___.__ or __ UNITS NO INSULIN DOSE REQUIRED FOR MEALS/SNACKS UNDER __G OF CARBS OR EQUAL TO __.__ OR LESS	TIME __:__ AM / PM LEFT ARM CGM / RIGHT ARM CGM / LEFT LEG CGM / RIGHT LEG CGM / LEFT/RIGHT STOMACH CGM KETONES NEGATIVE TRACE SMALL MODERATE LARGE
DINNER	Total Carbohydrates : ___._ grams	Correction Dose: (BS - ___) / __ (___-___)/__ = (__/__) = ___.__ Carb Dose Calculation: (Meal Carbs / ___) (__._ /___) = ___.__ Correction Dose + Carb Dose Calculation: (_____ + _____) = __.__ OR __ UNITS Correction Dose / Dose Calculation / Rounded to nearest whole number	TIME __:__ AM / PM LEFT ARM CGM / RIGHT ARM CGM / LEFT LEG CGM / RIGHT LEG CGM / LEFT/RIGHT STOMACH CGM KETONES NEGATIVE TRACE SMALL MODERATE LARGE
SNACK	Total Carbohydrates : ___._ grams	Carb Dose Calculation: (Meal Carbs / ___) (__._ /___) = ___.__ or __ UNITS NO INSULIN DOSE REQUIRED FOR MEALS/SNACKS UNDER __G OF CARBS OR EQUAL TO __.__ OR LESS	TIME __:__ AM / PM LEFT ARM CGM / RIGHT ARM CGM / LEFT LEG CGM / RIGHT LEG CGM / LEFT/RIGHT STOMACH CGM KETONES NEGATIVE TRACE SMALL MODERATE LARGE
BEDTIME __:__ PM	BLOOD SUGAR _____ UNITS ___ LEFT ARM CGM / RIGHT ARM CGM / LEFT LEG CGM / RIGHT LEG CGM / LEFT/RIGHT STOMACH CGM KETONES NEGATIVE TRACE SMALL MODERATE LARGE	HYDRATE 2AM BLOOD SUGAR _____ ADDITIONAL BLOOD SUGAR READINGS BS ___ at __ : __ AM/PM BS ___ at __ : __ AM/PM	NOTES MEDICINE

DATE: ____________________ SUN MON TUES WED THUR FRI SAT

	MEALS AND SNACKS	CARB AND FOOD CALCULATIONS	SHOT DETAILS AND LOCATION
BREAKFAST	Total Carbohydrates : ___._ grams	Correction Dose: (BS - ___) / __ (___-___)/__ = (__/__) = ___.__ Carb Dose Calculation: (Meal Carbs / ___) (__._ /___) = ___.__ Correction Dose + Carb Dose Calculation: (__.__ + __.__) = __.__ OR __ UNITS Correction Dose / Dose Calculation / Rounded to nearest whole number	TIME __ : __ AM / PM LEFT ARM CGM / RIGHT ARM CGM / LEFT LEG CGM / RIGHT LEG CGM / LEFT/RIGHT STOMACH CGM KETONES NEGATIVE TRACE SMALL MODERATE LARGE
SNACK	Total Carbohydrates : ___._ grams	Carb Dose Calculation: (Meal Carbs / ___) (__._ /___) = ___.__ or __ UNITS NO INSULIN DOSE REQUIRED FOR MEALS/SNACKS UNDER __G OF CARBS OR EQUAL TO __.__ OR LESS	TIME __ : __ AM / PM LEFT ARM CGM / RIGHT ARM CGM / LEFT LEG CGM / RIGHT LEG CGM / LEFT/RIGHT STOMACH CGM KETONES NEGATIVE TRACE SMALL MODERATE LARGE
LUNCH	Total Carbohydrates : ___._ grams	Correction Dose: (BS - ___) / __ (___-___)/__ = (__/__) = ___.__ Carb Dose Calculation: (Meal Carbs / ___) (__._ /___) = ___.__ Correction Dose + Carb Dose Calculation: (__.__ + __.__) = __.__ OR __ UNITS Correction Dose / Dose Calculation / Rounded to nearest whole number	TIME __ : __ AM / PM LEFT ARM CGM / RIGHT ARM CGM / LEFT LEG CGM / RIGHT LEG CGM / LEFT/RIGHT STOMACH CGM KETONES NEGATIVE TRACE SMALL MODERATE LARGE
SNACK	Total Carbohydrates : ___._ grams	Carb Dose Calculation: (Meal Carbs / ___) (__._ /___) = ___.__ or __ UNITS NO INSULIN DOSE REQUIRED FOR MEALS/SNACKS UNDER __G OF CARBS OR EQUAL TO __.__ OR LESS	TIME __ : __ AM / PM LEFT ARM CGM / RIGHT ARM CGM / LEFT LEG CGM / RIGHT LEG CGM / LEFT/RIGHT STOMACH CGM KETONES NEGATIVE TRACE SMALL MODERATE LARGE
DINNER	Total Carbohydrates : ___._ grams	Correction Dose: (BS - ___) / __ (___-___)/__ = (__/__) = ___.__ Carb Dose Calculation: (Meal Carbs / ___) (__._ /___) = ___.__ Correction Dose + Carb Dose Calculation: (__.__ + __.__) = __.__ OR __ UNITS Correction Dose / Dose Calculation / Rounded to nearest whole number	TIME __ : __ AM / PM LEFT ARM CGM / RIGHT ARM CGM / LEFT LEG CGM / RIGHT LEG CGM / LEFT/RIGHT STOMACH CGM KETONES NEGATIVE TRACE SMALL MODERATE LARGE
SNACK	Total Carbohydrates : ___._ grams	Carb Dose Calculation: (Meal Carbs / ___) (__._ /___) = ___.__ or __ UNITS NO INSULIN DOSE REQUIRED FOR MEALS/SNACKS UNDER __G OF CARBS OR EQUAL TO __.__ OR LESS	TIME __ : __ AM / PM LEFT ARM CGM / RIGHT ARM CGM / LEFT LEG CGM / RIGHT LEG CGM / LEFT/RIGHT STOMACH CGM KETONES NEGATIVE TRACE SMALL MODERATE LARGE
BEDTIME __ : __ PM	BLOOD SUGAR ____ UNITS ___ LEFT ARM CGM / RIGHT ARM CGM / LEFT LEG CGM / RIGHT LEG CGM / LEFT/RIGHT STOMACH CGM KETONES NEGATIVE TRACE SMALL MODERATE LARGE	HYDRATE 2AM BLOOD SUGAR ____ ADDITIONAL BLOOD SUGAR READINGS BS ___ at __ : __ AM/PM BS ___ at __ : __ AM/PM	NOTES MEDICINE

DATE: ______________________ SUN MON TUES WED THUR FRI SAT

	MEALS AND SNACKS	CARB AND FOOD CALCULATIONS	SHOT DETAILS AND LOCATION
BREAKFAST	Total Carbohydrates : ___._ grams	Correction Dose: (BS - ___) / __ (___-___)/__ = (__/__) = ___.__ Carb Dose Calculation: (Meal Carbs / ___) (__._ /___) = ___.__ Correction Dose + Carb Dose Calculation: (___.__ + ___.__) = __.__ OR __ UNITS Correction Dose / Dose Calculation / Rounded to nearest whole number	TIME __ :__ AM / PM LEFT ARM CGM / RIGHT ARM CGM / LEFT LEG CGM / RIGHT LEG CGM / LEFT/RIGHT STOMACH CGM KETONES NEGATIVE / TRACE / SMALL / MODERATE / LARGE
SNACK	Total Carbohydrates : ___._ grams	Carb Dose Calculation: (Meal Carbs / ___) (__._ /___) = ___.__ or __ UNITS NO INSULIN DOSE REQUIRED FOR MEALS/SNACKS UNDER __G OF CARBS OR EQUAL TO __.__ OR LESS	TIME __ :__ AM / PM LEFT ARM CGM / RIGHT ARM CGM / LEFT LEG CGM / RIGHT LEG CGM / LEFT/RIGHT STOMACH CGM KETONES NEGATIVE / TRACE / SMALL / MODERATE / LARGE
LUNCH	Total Carbohydrates : ___._ grams	Correction Dose: (BS - ___) / __ (___-___)/__ = (__/__) = ___.__ Carb Dose Calculation: (Meal Carbs / ___) (__._ /___) = ___.__ Correction Dose + Carb Dose Calculation: (___.__ + ___.__) = __.__ OR __ UNITS Correction Dose / Dose Calculation / Rounded to nearest whole number	TIME __ :__ AM / PM LEFT ARM CGM / RIGHT ARM CGM / LEFT LEG CGM / RIGHT LEG CGM / LEFT/RIGHT STOMACH CGM KETONES NEGATIVE / TRACE / SMALL / MODERATE / LARGE
SNACK	Total Carbohydrates : ___._ grams	Carb Dose Calculation: (Meal Carbs / ___) (__._ /___) = ___.__ or __ UNITS NO INSULIN DOSE REQUIRED FOR MEALS/SNACKS UNDER __G OF CARBS OR EQUAL TO __.__ OR LESS	TIME __ :__ AM / PM LEFT ARM CGM / RIGHT ARM CGM / LEFT LEG CGM / RIGHT LEG CGM / LEFT/RIGHT STOMACH CGM KETONES NEGATIVE / TRACE / SMALL / MODERATE / LARGE
DINNER	Total Carbohydrates : ___._ grams	Correction Dose: (BS - ___) / __ (___-___)/__ = (__/__) = ___.__ Carb Dose Calculation: (Meal Carbs / ___) (__._ /___) = ___.__ Correction Dose + Carb Dose Calculation: (___.__ + ___.__) = __.__ OR __ UNITS Correction Dose / Dose Calculation / Rounded to nearest whole number	TIME __ :__ AM / PM LEFT ARM CGM / RIGHT ARM CGM / LEFT LEG CGM / RIGHT LEG CGM / LEFT/RIGHT STOMACH CGM KETONES NEGATIVE / TRACE / SMALL / MODERATE / LARGE
SNACK	Total Carbohydrates : ___._ grams	Carb Dose Calculation: (Meal Carbs / ___) (__._ /___) = ___.__ or __ UNITS NO INSULIN DOSE REQUIRED FOR MEALS/SNACKS UNDER __G OF CARBS OR EQUAL TO __.__ OR LESS	TIME __ :__ AM / PM LEFT ARM CGM / RIGHT ARM CGM / LEFT LEG CGM / RIGHT LEG CGM / LEFT/RIGHT STOMACH CGM KETONES NEGATIVE / TRACE / SMALL / MODERATE / LARGE
BEDTIME __ : __ PM	BLOOD SUGAR _____ UNITS ___ LEFT ARM CGM / RIGHT ARM CGM / LEFT LEG CGM / RIGHT LEG CGM / LEFT/RIGHT STOMACH CGM KETONES NEGATIVE / TRACE / SMALL / MODERATE / LARGE	HYDRATE 2AM BLOOD SUGAR _____ ADDITIONAL BLOOD SUGAR READINGS BS ___ at __ : __ AM/PM BS ___ at __ : __ AM/PM	NOTES MEDICINE

DATE: ______________________ SUN MON TUES WED THUR FRI SAT

	MEALS AND SNACKS	CARB AND FOOD CALCULATIONS	SHOT DETAILS AND LOCATION
BREAKFAST	Total Carbohydrates : ___._ grams	Correction Dose: (BS - ___) / __ (___-___)/__ = (__/__) = ___.__ Carb Dose Calculation: (Meal Carbs / ___) (__._ /___) = ___.__ Correction Dose + Carb Dose Calculation: (__.__ + __.__) = __.__ OR __ UNITS Correction Dose / Dose Calculation / Rounded to nearest whole number	TIME __ : __ AM / PM LEFT ARM CGM / RIGHT ARM CGM / LEFT LEG CGM / RIGHT LEG CGM / LEFT/RIGHT STOMACH CGM KETONES NEGATIVE / TRACE / SMALL / MODERATE / LARGE
SNACK	Total Carbohydrates : ___._ grams	Carb Dose Calculation: (Meal Carbs / ___) (__._ /___) = ___.__ or __ UNITS NO INSULIN DOSE REQUIRED FOR MEALS/SNACKS UNDER __G OF CARBS OR EQUAL TO __.__ OR LESS	TIME __ : __ AM / PM LEFT ARM CGM / RIGHT ARM CGM / LEFT LEG CGM / RIGHT LEG CGM / LEFT/RIGHT STOMACH CGM KETONES NEGATIVE / TRACE / SMALL / MODERATE / LARGE
LUNCH	Total Carbohydrates : ___._ grams	Correction Dose: (BS - ___) / __ (___-___)/__ = (__/__) = ___.__ Carb Dose Calculation: (Meal Carbs / ___) (__._ /___) = ___.__ Correction Dose + Carb Dose Calculation: (__.__ + __.__) = __.__ OR __ UNITS Correction Dose / Dose Calculation / Rounded to nearest whole number	TIME __ : __ AM / PM LEFT ARM CGM / RIGHT ARM CGM / LEFT LEG CGM / RIGHT LEG CGM / LEFT/RIGHT STOMACH CGM KETONES NEGATIVE / TRACE / SMALL / MODERATE / LARGE
SNACK	Total Carbohydrates : ___._ grams	Carb Dose Calculation: (Meal Carbs / ___) (__._ /___) = ___.__ or __ UNITS NO INSULIN DOSE REQUIRED FOR MEALS/SNACKS UNDER __G OF CARBS OR EQUAL TO __.__ OR LESS	TIME __ : __ AM / PM LEFT ARM CGM / RIGHT ARM CGM / LEFT LEG CGM / RIGHT LEG CGM / LEFT/RIGHT STOMACH CGM KETONES NEGATIVE / TRACE / SMALL / MODERATE / LARGE
DINNER	Total Carbohydrates : ___._ grams	Correction Dose: (BS - ___) / __ (___-___)/__ = (__/__) = ___.__ Carb Dose Calculation: (Meal Carbs / ___) (__._ /___) = ___.__ Correction Dose + Carb Dose Calculation: (__.__ + __.__) = __.__ OR __ UNITS Correction Dose / Dose Calculation / Rounded to nearest whole number	TIME __ : __ AM / PM LEFT ARM CGM / RIGHT ARM CGM / LEFT LEG CGM / RIGHT LEG CGM / LEFT/RIGHT STOMACH CGM KETONES NEGATIVE / TRACE / SMALL / MODERATE / LARGE
SNACK	Total Carbohydrates : ___._ grams	Carb Dose Calculation: (Meal Carbs / ___) (__._ /___) = ___.__ or __ UNITS NO INSULIN DOSE REQUIRED FOR MEALS/SNACKS UNDER __G OF CARBS OR EQUAL TO __.__ OR LESS	TIME __ : __ AM / PM LEFT ARM CGM / RIGHT ARM CGM / LEFT LEG CGM / RIGHT LEG CGM / LEFT/RIGHT STOMACH CGM KETONES NEGATIVE / TRACE / SMALL / MODERATE / LARGE
BEDTIME __ : __ PM	BLOOD SUGAR _____ UNITS ___ LEFT ARM CGM / RIGHT ARM CGM / LEFT LEG CGM / RIGHT LEG CGM / LEFT/RIGHT STOMACH CGM KETONES NEGATIVE / TRACE / SMALL / MODERATE / LARGE	HYDRATE 2AM BLOOD SUGAR _____ ADDITIONAL BLOOD SUGAR READINGS BS ___ at __ : __ AM/PM BS ___ at __ : __ AM/PM	NOTES MEDICINE

DATE: ____________________ SUN MON TUES WED THUR FRI SAT

	MEALS AND SNACKS	CARB AND FOOD CALCULATIONS	SHOT DETAILS AND LOCATION
BREAKFAST	Total Carbohydrates : ___._ grams	Correction Dose: (BS - ___) / __ (___-___)/__ = (__/__) = ___.__ Carb Dose Calculation: (Meal Carbs / ___) (__._ /___) = ___.__ Correction Dose + Carb Dose Calculation: (______ + ______) = __.__ OR __ UNITS Correction Dose · Dose Calculation · Rounded to nearest whole number	TIME __ : __ AM / PM LEFT ARM CGM · RIGHT ARM CGM · LEFT LEG CGM · RIGHT LEG CGM · LEFT/RIGHT STOMACH CGM KETONES NEGATIVE · TRACE · SMALL · MODERATE · LARGE
SNACK	Total Carbohydrates : ___._ grams	Carb Dose Calculation: (Meal Carbs / ___) (__._ /___) = ___.__ or __ UNITS NO INSULIN DOSE REQUIRED FOR MEALS/SNACKS UNDER __G OF CARBS OR EQUAL TO __.__ OR LESS	TIME __ : __ AM / PM LEFT ARM CGM · RIGHT ARM CGM · LEFT LEG CGM · RIGHT LEG CGM · LEFT/RIGHT STOMACH CGM KETONES NEGATIVE · TRACE · SMALL · MODERATE · LARGE
LUNCH	Total Carbohydrates : ___._ grams	Correction Dose: (BS - ___) / __ (___-___)/__ = (__/__) = ___.__ Carb Dose Calculation: (Meal Carbs / ___) (__._ /___) = ___.__ Correction Dose + Carb Dose Calculation: (______ + ______) = __.__ OR __ UNITS Correction Dose · Dose Calculation · Rounded to nearest whole number	TIME __ : __ AM / PM LEFT ARM CGM · RIGHT ARM CGM · LEFT LEG CGM · RIGHT LEG CGM · LEFT/RIGHT STOMACH CGM KETONES NEGATIVE · TRACE · SMALL · MODERATE · LARGE
SNACK	Total Carbohydrates : ___._ grams	Carb Dose Calculation: (Meal Carbs / ___) (__._ /___) = ___.__ or __ UNITS NO INSULIN DOSE REQUIRED FOR MEALS/SNACKS UNDER __G OF CARBS OR EQUAL TO __.__ OR LESS	TIME __ : __ AM / PM LEFT ARM CGM · RIGHT ARM CGM · LEFT LEG CGM · RIGHT LEG CGM · LEFT/RIGHT STOMACH CGM KETONES NEGATIVE · TRACE · SMALL · MODERATE · LARGE
DINNER	Total Carbohydrates : ___._ grams	Correction Dose: (BS - ___) / __ (___-___)/__ = (__/__) = ___.__ Carb Dose Calculation: (Meal Carbs / ___) (__._ /___) = ___.__ Correction Dose + Carb Dose Calculation: (______ + ______) = __.__ OR __ UNITS Correction Dose · Dose Calculation · Rounded to nearest whole number	TIME __ : __ AM / PM LEFT ARM CGM · RIGHT ARM CGM · LEFT LEG CGM · RIGHT LEG CGM · LEFT/RIGHT STOMACH CGM KETONES NEGATIVE · TRACE · SMALL · MODERATE · LARGE
SNACK	Total Carbohydrates : ___._ grams	Carb Dose Calculation: (Meal Carbs / ___) (__._ /___) = ___.__ or __ UNITS NO INSULIN DOSE REQUIRED FOR MEALS/SNACKS UNDER __G OF CARBS OR EQUAL TO __.__ OR LESS	TIME __ : __ AM / PM LEFT ARM CGM · RIGHT ARM CGM · LEFT LEG CGM · RIGHT LEG CGM · LEFT/RIGHT STOMACH CGM KETONES NEGATIVE · TRACE · SMALL · MODERATE · LARGE
BEDTIME __ : __ PM	BLOOD SUGAR ____ UNITS ___ LEFT ARM CGM · RIGHT ARM CGM · LEFT LEG CGM · RIGHT LEG CGM · LEFT/RIGHT STOMACH CGM KETONES NEGATIVE · TRACE · SMALL · MODERATE · LARGE	HYDRATE 2AM BLOOD SUGAR ____ ADDITIONAL BLOOD SUGAR READINGS BS ___ at __ : __ AM/PM BS ___ at __ : __ AM/PM	NOTES MEDICINE

DATE: ______________________ SUN MON TUES WED THUR FRI SAT

	MEALS AND SNACKS	CARB AND FOOD CALCULATIONS	SHOT DETAILS AND LOCATION
BREAKFAST	Total Carbohydrates : ___._ grams	Correction Dose: (BS - ___) / __ (___-___)/__ = (__/__) = ___.__ Carb Dose Calculation: (Meal Carbs / ___) (__._ /___) = ___.__ Correction Dose + Carb Dose Calculation: (___.__ + ___.__) = __.__ OR __ UNITS Correction Dose / Dose Calculation / Rounded to nearest whole number	TIME __ : __ AM / PM LEFT ARM CGM / RIGHT ARM CGM / LEFT LEG CGM / RIGHT LEG CGM / LEFT/RIGHT STOMACH CGM KETONES NEGATIVE / TRACE / SMALL / MODERATE / LARGE
SNACK	Total Carbohydrates : ___._ grams	Carb Dose Calculation: (Meal Carbs / ___) (__._ /___) = ___.__ or __ UNITS NO INSULIN DOSE REQUIRED FOR MEALS/SNACKS UNDER __G OF CARBS OR EQUAL TO __.__ OR LESS	TIME __ : __ AM / PM LEFT ARM CGM / RIGHT ARM CGM / LEFT LEG CGM / RIGHT LEG CGM / LEFT/RIGHT STOMACH CGM KETONES NEGATIVE / TRACE / SMALL / MODERATE / LARGE
LUNCH	Total Carbohydrates : ___._ grams	Correction Dose: (BS - ___) / __ (___-___)/__ = (__/__) = ___.__ Carb Dose Calculation: (Meal Carbs / ___) (__._ /___) = ___.__ Correction Dose + Carb Dose Calculation: (___.__ + ___.__) = __.__ OR __ UNITS Correction Dose / Dose Calculation / Rounded to nearest whole number	TIME __ : __ AM / PM LEFT ARM CGM / RIGHT ARM CGM / LEFT LEG CGM / RIGHT LEG CGM / LEFT/RIGHT STOMACH CGM KETONES NEGATIVE / TRACE / SMALL / MODERATE / LARGE
SNACK	Total Carbohydrates : ___._ grams	Carb Dose Calculation: (Meal Carbs / ___) (__._ /___) = ___.__ or __ UNITS NO INSULIN DOSE REQUIRED FOR MEALS/SNACKS UNDER __G OF CARBS OR EQUAL TO __.__ OR LESS	TIME __ : __ AM / PM LEFT ARM CGM / RIGHT ARM CGM / LEFT LEG CGM / RIGHT LEG CGM / LEFT/RIGHT STOMACH CGM KETONES NEGATIVE / TRACE / SMALL / MODERATE / LARGE
DINNER	Total Carbohydrates : ___._ grams	Correction Dose: (BS - ___) / __ (___-___)/__ = (__/__) = ___.__ Carb Dose Calculation: (Meal Carbs / ___) (__._ /___) = ___.__ Correction Dose + Carb Dose Calculation: (___.__ + ___.__) = __.__ OR __ UNITS Correction Dose / Dose Calculation / Rounded to nearest whole number	TIME __ : __ AM / PM LEFT ARM CGM / RIGHT ARM CGM / LEFT LEG CGM / RIGHT LEG CGM / LEFT/RIGHT STOMACH CGM KETONES NEGATIVE / TRACE / SMALL / MODERATE / LARGE
SNACK	Total Carbohydrates : ___._ grams	Carb Dose Calculation: (Meal Carbs / ___) (__._ /___) = ___.__ or __ UNITS NO INSULIN DOSE REQUIRED FOR MEALS/SNACKS UNDER __G OF CARBS OR EQUAL TO __.__ OR LESS	TIME __ : __ AM / PM LEFT ARM CGM / RIGHT ARM CGM / LEFT LEG CGM / RIGHT LEG CGM / LEFT/RIGHT STOMACH CGM KETONES NEGATIVE / TRACE / SMALL / MODERATE / LARGE
BEDTIME __ : __ PM	BLOOD SUGAR _____ UNITS ___ LEFT ARM CGM / RIGHT ARM CGM / LEFT LEG CGM / RIGHT LEG CGM / LEFT/RIGHT STOMACH CGM KETONES NEGATIVE / TRACE / SMALL / MODERATE / LARGE	HYDRATE 2AM BLOOD SUGAR _____ ADDITIONAL BLOOD SUGAR READINGS BS ___ at __ : __ AM/PM BS ___ at __ : __ AM/PM	NOTES MEDICINE

DATE: ______________________ SUN MON TUES WED THUR FRI SAT

	MEALS AND SNACKS	CARB AND FOOD CALCULATIONS	SHOT DETAILS AND LOCATION
BREAKFAST	Total Carbohydrates : ___._ grams	Correction Dose: (BS - ___) / __ (___-___)/__ = (__/__) = ___.__ Carb Dose Calculation: (Meal Carbs / ___) (__._ /___) = ___.__ Correction Dose + Carb Dose Calculation: (_____ + _____) = __.__ OR __ UNITS Correction Dose / Dose Calculation / Rounded to nearest whole number	TIME __ : __ AM / PM LEFT ARM CGM / RIGHT ARM CGM / LEFT LEG CGM / RIGHT LEG CGM / LEFT/RIGHT STOMACH CGM KETONES NEGATIVE TRACE SMALL MODERATE LARGE
SNACK	Total Carbohydrates : ___._ grams	Carb Dose Calculation: (Meal Carbs / ___) (__._ /___) = ___.__ or __ UNITS NO INSULIN DOSE REQUIRED FOR MEALS/SNACKS UNDER __G OF CARBS OR EQUAL TO __.__ OR LESS	TIME __ : __ AM / PM LEFT ARM CGM / RIGHT ARM CGM / LEFT LEG CGM / RIGHT LEG CGM / LEFT/RIGHT STOMACH CGM KETONES NEGATIVE TRACE SMALL MODERATE LARGE
LUNCH	Total Carbohydrates : ___._ grams	Correction Dose: (BS - ___) / __ (___-___)/__ = (__/__) = ___.__ Carb Dose Calculation: (Meal Carbs / ___) (__._ /___) = ___.__ Correction Dose + Carb Dose Calculation: (_____ + _____) = __.__ OR __ UNITS Correction Dose / Dose Calculation / Rounded to nearest whole number	TIME __ : __ AM / PM LEFT ARM CGM / RIGHT ARM CGM / LEFT LEG CGM / RIGHT LEG CGM / LEFT/RIGHT STOMACH CGM KETONES NEGATIVE TRACE SMALL MODERATE LARGE
SNACK	Total Carbohydrates : ___._ grams	Carb Dose Calculation: (Meal Carbs / ___) (__._ /___) = ___.__ or __ UNITS NO INSULIN DOSE REQUIRED FOR MEALS/SNACKS UNDER __G OF CARBS OR EQUAL TO __.__ OR LESS	TIME __ : __ AM / PM LEFT ARM CGM / RIGHT ARM CGM / LEFT LEG CGM / RIGHT LEG CGM / LEFT/RIGHT STOMACH CGM KETONES NEGATIVE TRACE SMALL MODERATE LARGE
DINNER	Total Carbohydrates : ___._ grams	Correction Dose: (BS - ___) / __ (___-___)/__ = (__/__) = ___.__ Carb Dose Calculation: (Meal Carbs / ___) (__._ /___) = ___.__ Correction Dose + Carb Dose Calculation: (_____ + _____) = __.__ OR __ UNITS Correction Dose / Dose Calculation / Rounded to nearest whole number	TIME __ : __ AM / PM LEFT ARM CGM / RIGHT ARM CGM / LEFT LEG CGM / RIGHT LEG CGM / LEFT/RIGHT STOMACH CGM KETONES NEGATIVE TRACE SMALL MODERATE LARGE
SNACK	Total Carbohydrates : ___._ grams	Carb Dose Calculation: (Meal Carbs / ___) (__._ /___) = ___.__ or __ UNITS NO INSULIN DOSE REQUIRED FOR MEALS/SNACKS UNDER __G OF CARBS OR EQUAL TO __.__ OR LESS	TIME __ : __ AM / PM LEFT ARM CGM / RIGHT ARM CGM / LEFT LEG CGM / RIGHT LEG CGM / LEFT/RIGHT STOMACH CGM KETONES NEGATIVE TRACE SMALL MODERATE LARGE
BEDTIME __ : __ PM	BLOOD SUGAR ____ UNITS ___ LEFT ARM CGM / RIGHT ARM CGM / LEFT LEG CGM / RIGHT LEG CGM / LEFT/RIGHT STOMACH CGM KETONES NEGATIVE TRACE SMALL MODERATE LARGE	HYDRATE 2AM BLOOD SUGAR ____ ADDITIONAL BLOOD SUGAR READINGS BS ___ at __ : __ AM/PM BS ___ at __ : __ AM/PM	NOTES MEDICINE

DATE: ______________________________ SUN MON TUES WED THUR FRI SAT

	MEALS AND SNACKS	CARB AND FOOD CALCULATIONS	SHOT DETAILS AND LOCATION
BREAKFAST	Total Carbohydrates : ___._ grams	Correction Dose: (BS - ___) / __ (___-___)/__ = (__/__) = ___.__ Carb Dose Calculation: (Meal Carbs / ___) (__._ /___) = ___.__ Correction Dose + Carb Dose Calculation: (__.__ + __.__) = __.__ OR __ UNITS Correction Dose / Dose Calculation / Rounded to nearest whole number	TIME __ : __ AM / PM LEFT ARM CGM / RIGHT ARM CGM / LEFT LEG CGM / RIGHT LEG CGM / LEFT/RIGHT STOMACH CGM KETONES NEGATIVE TRACE SMALL MODERATE LARGE
SNACK	Total Carbohydrates : ___._ grams	Carb Dose Calculation: (Meal Carbs / ___) (__._ /___) = ___.__ or __ UNITS NO INSULIN DOSE REQUIRED FOR MEALS/SNACKS UNDER __G OF CARBS OR EQUAL TO __.__ OR LESS	TIME __ : __ AM / PM LEFT ARM CGM / RIGHT ARM CGM / LEFT LEG CGM / RIGHT LEG CGM / LEFT/RIGHT STOMACH CGM KETONES NEGATIVE TRACE SMALL MODERATE LARGE
LUNCH	Total Carbohydrates : ___._ grams	Correction Dose: (BS - ___) / __ (___-___)/__ = (__/__) = ___.__ Carb Dose Calculation: (Meal Carbs / ___) (__._ /___) = ___.__ Correction Dose + Carb Dose Calculation: (__.__ + __.__) = __.__ OR __ UNITS Correction Dose / Dose Calculation / Rounded to nearest whole number	TIME __ : __ AM / PM LEFT ARM CGM / RIGHT ARM CGM / LEFT LEG CGM / RIGHT LEG CGM / LEFT/RIGHT STOMACH CGM KETONES NEGATIVE TRACE SMALL MODERATE LARGE
SNACK	Total Carbohydrates : ___._ grams	Carb Dose Calculation: (Meal Carbs / ___) (__._ /___) = ___.__ or __ UNITS NO INSULIN DOSE REQUIRED FOR MEALS/SNACKS UNDER __G OF CARBS OR EQUAL TO __.__ OR LESS	TIME __ : __ AM / PM LEFT ARM CGM / RIGHT ARM CGM / LEFT LEG CGM / RIGHT LEG CGM / LEFT/RIGHT STOMACH CGM KETONES NEGATIVE TRACE SMALL MODERATE LARGE
DINNER	Total Carbohydrates : ___._ grams	Correction Dose: (BS - ___) / __ (___-___)/__ = (__/__) = ___.__ Carb Dose Calculation: (Meal Carbs / ___) (__._ /___) = ___.__ Correction Dose + Carb Dose Calculation: (__.__ + __.__) = __.__ OR __ UNITS Correction Dose / Dose Calculation / Rounded to nearest whole number	TIME __ : __ AM / PM LEFT ARM CGM / RIGHT ARM CGM / LEFT LEG CGM / RIGHT LEG CGM / LEFT/RIGHT STOMACH CGM KETONES NEGATIVE TRACE SMALL MODERATE LARGE
SNACK	Total Carbohydrates : ___._ grams	Carb Dose Calculation: (Meal Carbs / ___) (__._ /___) = ___.__ or __ UNITS NO INSULIN DOSE REQUIRED FOR MEALS/SNACKS UNDER __G OF CARBS OR EQUAL TO __.__ OR LESS	TIME __ : __ AM / PM LEFT ARM CGM / RIGHT ARM CGM / LEFT LEG CGM / RIGHT LEG CGM / LEFT/RIGHT STOMACH CGM KETONES NEGATIVE TRACE SMALL MODERATE LARGE
BEDTIME __ : __ PM	BLOOD SUGAR _____ UNITS ___ LEFT ARM CGM / RIGHT ARM CGM / LEFT LEG CGM / RIGHT LEG CGM / LEFT/RIGHT STOMACH CGM KETONES NEGATIVE TRACE SMALL MODERATE LARGE	HYDRATE 2AM BLOOD SUGAR _____ ADDITIONAL BLOOD SUGAR READINGS BS ___ at __ : __ AM/PM BS ___ at __ : __ AM/PM	NOTES MEDICINE

DATE: ______________________ SUN MON TUES WED THUR FRI SAT

	MEALS AND SNACKS	CARB AND FOOD CALCULATIONS	SHOT DETAILS AND LOCATION
BREAKFAST	Total Carbohydrates : ___._ grams	Correction Dose: (BS - ___) / __ (___-___)/__ = (__/__) = ___.__ Carb Dose Calculation: (Meal Carbs / ___) (__._ /___) = ___.__ Correction Dose + Carb Dose Calculation: (_____ + _____) = __.__ OR __ UNITS Correction Dose Dose Calculation Rounded to nearest whole number	TIME __ : __ AM / PM LEFT ARM CGM | RIGHT ARM CGM | LEFT LEG CGM | RIGHT LEG CGM | LEFT/RIGHT STOMACH CGM KETONES NEGATIVE TRACE SMALL MODERATE LARGE
SNACK	Total Carbohydrates : ___._ grams	Carb Dose Calculation: (Meal Carbs / ___) (__._ /___) = ___.__ or __ UNITS NO INSULIN DOSE REQUIRED FOR MEALS/SNACKS UNDER __G OF CARBS OR EQUAL TO __.__ OR LESS	TIME __ : __ AM / PM LEFT ARM CGM | RIGHT ARM CGM | LEFT LEG CGM | RIGHT LEG CGM | LEFT/RIGHT STOMACH CGM KETONES NEGATIVE TRACE SMALL MODERATE LARGE
LUNCH	Total Carbohydrates : ___._ grams	Correction Dose: (BS - ___) / __ (___-___)/__ = (__/__) = ___.__ Carb Dose Calculation: (Meal Carbs / ___) (__._ /___) = ___.__ Correction Dose + Carb Dose Calculation: (_____ + _____) = __.__ OR __ UNITS Correction Dose Dose Calculation Rounded to nearest whole number	TIME __ : __ AM / PM LEFT ARM CGM | RIGHT ARM CGM | LEFT LEG CGM | RIGHT LEG CGM | LEFT/RIGHT STOMACH CGM KETONES NEGATIVE TRACE SMALL MODERATE LARGE
SNACK	Total Carbohydrates : ___._ grams	Carb Dose Calculation: (Meal Carbs / ___) (__._ /___) = ___.__ or __ UNITS NO INSULIN DOSE REQUIRED FOR MEALS/SNACKS UNDER __G OF CARBS OR EQUAL TO __.__ OR LESS	TIME __ : __ AM / PM LEFT ARM CGM | RIGHT ARM CGM | LEFT LEG CGM | RIGHT LEG CGM | LEFT/RIGHT STOMACH CGM KETONES NEGATIVE TRACE SMALL MODERATE LARGE
DINNER	Total Carbohydrates : ___._ grams	Correction Dose: (BS - ___) / __ (___-___)/__ = (__/__) = ___.__ Carb Dose Calculation: (Meal Carbs / ___) (__._ /___) = ___.__ Correction Dose + Carb Dose Calculation: (_____ + _____) = __.__ OR __ UNITS Correction Dose Dose Calculation Rounded to nearest whole number	TIME __ : __ AM / PM LEFT ARM CGM | RIGHT ARM CGM | LEFT LEG CGM | RIGHT LEG CGM | LEFT/RIGHT STOMACH CGM KETONES NEGATIVE TRACE SMALL MODERATE LARGE
SNACK	Total Carbohydrates : ___._ grams	Carb Dose Calculation: (Meal Carbs / ___) (__._ /___) = ___.__ or __ UNITS NO INSULIN DOSE REQUIRED FOR MEALS/SNACKS UNDER __G OF CARBS OR EQUAL TO __.__ OR LESS	TIME __ : __ AM / PM LEFT ARM CGM | RIGHT ARM CGM | LEFT LEG CGM | RIGHT LEG CGM | LEFT/RIGHT STOMACH CGM KETONES NEGATIVE TRACE SMALL MODERATE LARGE
BEDTIME __ : __ PM	BLOOD SUGAR ____ UNITS ___ LEFT ARM CGM | RIGHT ARM CGM | LEFT LEG CGM | RIGHT LEG CGM | LEFT/RIGHT STOMACH CGM KETONES NEGATIVE TRACE SMALL MODERATE LARGE	HYDRATE 2AM BLOOD SUGAR ____ ADDITIONAL BLOOD SUGAR READINGS BS ___ at __ : __ AM/PM BS ___ at __ : __ AM/PM	NOTES MEDICINE

DATE: ______________________________ SUN MON TUES WED THUR FRI SAT

	MEALS AND SNACKS	CARB AND FOOD CALCULATIONS	SHOT DETAILS AND LOCATION
BREAKFAST	Total Carbohydrates : ___._ grams	Correction Dose: (BS - ___) / __ (___-___)/__ = (__/__) = ___.__ Carb Dose Calculation: (Meal Carbs / ___) (__._ /___) = ___.__ Correction Dose + Carb Dose Calculation: (__.__ + __.__) = __.__ OR __ UNITS Correction Dose / Dose Calculation / Rounded to nearest whole number	TIME __ : __ AM / PM LEFT ARM CGM / RIGHT ARM CGM / LEFT LEG CGM / RIGHT LEG CGM / LEFT/RIGHT STOMACH CGM KETONES NEGATIVE / TRACE / SMALL / MODERATE / LARGE
SNACK	Total Carbohydrates : ___._ grams	Carb Dose Calculation: (Meal Carbs / ___) (__._ /___) = ___.__ or __ UNITS NO INSULIN DOSE REQUIRED FOR MEALS/SNACKS UNDER __G OF CARBS OR EQUAL TO __.__ OR LESS	TIME __ : __ AM / PM LEFT ARM CGM / RIGHT ARM CGM / LEFT LEG CGM / RIGHT LEG CGM / LEFT/RIGHT STOMACH CGM KETONES NEGATIVE / TRACE / SMALL / MODERATE / LARGE
LUNCH	Total Carbohydrates : ___._ grams	Correction Dose: (BS - ___) / __ (___-___)/__ = (__/__) = ___.__ Carb Dose Calculation: (Meal Carbs / ___) (__._ /___) = ___.__ Correction Dose + Carb Dose Calculation: (__.__ + __.__) = __.__ OR __ UNITS Correction Dose / Dose Calculation / Rounded to nearest whole number	TIME __ : __ AM / PM LEFT ARM CGM / RIGHT ARM CGM / LEFT LEG CGM / RIGHT LEG CGM / LEFT/RIGHT STOMACH CGM KETONES NEGATIVE / TRACE / SMALL / MODERATE / LARGE
SNACK	Total Carbohydrates : ___._ grams	Carb Dose Calculation: (Meal Carbs / ___) (__._ /___) = ___.__ or __ UNITS NO INSULIN DOSE REQUIRED FOR MEALS/SNACKS UNDER __G OF CARBS OR EQUAL TO __.__ OR LESS	TIME __ : __ AM / PM LEFT ARM CGM / RIGHT ARM CGM / LEFT LEG CGM / RIGHT LEG CGM / LEFT/RIGHT STOMACH CGM KETONES NEGATIVE / TRACE / SMALL / MODERATE / LARGE
DINNER	Total Carbohydrates : ___._ grams	Correction Dose: (BS - ___) / __ (___-___)/__ = (__/__) = ___.__ Carb Dose Calculation: (Meal Carbs / ___) (__._ /___) = ___.__ Correction Dose + Carb Dose Calculation: (__.__ + __.__) = __.__ OR __ UNITS Correction Dose / Dose Calculation / Rounded to nearest whole number	TIME __ : __ AM / PM LEFT ARM CGM / RIGHT ARM CGM / LEFT LEG CGM / RIGHT LEG CGM / LEFT/RIGHT STOMACH CGM KETONES NEGATIVE / TRACE / SMALL / MODERATE / LARGE
SNACK	Total Carbohydrates : ___._ grams	Carb Dose Calculation: (Meal Carbs / ___) (__._ /___) = ___.__ or __ UNITS NO INSULIN DOSE REQUIRED FOR MEALS/SNACKS UNDER __G OF CARBS OR EQUAL TO __.__ OR LESS	TIME __ : __ AM / PM LEFT ARM CGM / RIGHT ARM CGM / LEFT LEG CGM / RIGHT LEG CGM / LEFT/RIGHT STOMACH CGM KETONES NEGATIVE / TRACE / SMALL / MODERATE / LARGE
BEDTIME __ : __ PM	BLOOD SUGAR ____ UNITS ___ LEFT ARM CGM / RIGHT ARM CGM / LEFT LEG CGM / RIGHT LEG CGM / LEFT/RIGHT STOMACH CGM KETONES NEGATIVE / TRACE / SMALL / MODERATE / LARGE	HYDRATE 2AM BLOOD SUGAR ____ ADDITIONAL BLOOD SUGAR READINGS BS ___ at __ : __ AM/PM BS ___ at __ : __ AM/PM	NOTES MEDICINE

DATE: ______________________ SUN MON TUES WED THUR FRI SAT

	MEALS AND SNACKS	CARB AND FOOD CALCULATIONS	SHOT DETAILS AND LOCATION
BREAKFAST	Total Carbohydrates : ___._ grams	Correction Dose: (BS - ___) / __ (___-___)/__ = (__/__) = ___.__ Carb Dose Calculation: (Meal Carbs / ___) (__._ /___) = ___.__ Correction Dose + Carb Dose Calculation: (_____ + _____) = __.__ OR __ UNITS Correction Dose / Dose Calculation / Rounded to nearest whole number	TIME __ :__ AM / PM LEFT ARM CGM / RIGHT ARM CGM / LEFT LEG CGM / RIGHT LEG CGM / LEFT/RIGHT STOMACH CGM KETONES NEGATIVE / TRACE / SMALL / MODERATE / LARGE
SNACK	Total Carbohydrates : ___._ grams	Carb Dose Calculation: (Meal Carbs / ___) (__._ /___) = ___.__ or __ UNITS NO INSULIN DOSE REQUIRED FOR MEALS/SNACKS UNDER __G OF CARBS OR EQUAL TO __.__ OR LESS	TIME __ :__ AM / PM LEFT ARM CGM / RIGHT ARM CGM / LEFT LEG CGM / RIGHT LEG CGM / LEFT/RIGHT STOMACH CGM KETONES NEGATIVE / TRACE / SMALL / MODERATE / LARGE
LUNCH	Total Carbohydrates : ___._ grams	Correction Dose: (BS - ___) / __ (___-___)/__ = (__/__) = ___.__ Carb Dose Calculation: (Meal Carbs / ___) (__._ /___) = ___.__ Correction Dose + Carb Dose Calculation: (_____ + _____) = __.__ OR __ UNITS Correction Dose / Dose Calculation / Rounded to nearest whole number	TIME __ :__ AM / PM LEFT ARM CGM / RIGHT ARM CGM / LEFT LEG CGM / RIGHT LEG CGM / LEFT/RIGHT STOMACH CGM KETONES NEGATIVE / TRACE / SMALL / MODERATE / LARGE
SNACK	Total Carbohydrates : ___._ grams	Carb Dose Calculation: (Meal Carbs / ___) (__._ /___) = ___.__ or __ UNITS NO INSULIN DOSE REQUIRED FOR MEALS/SNACKS UNDER __G OF CARBS OR EQUAL TO __.__ OR LESS	TIME __ :__ AM / PM LEFT ARM CGM / RIGHT ARM CGM / LEFT LEG CGM / RIGHT LEG CGM / LEFT/RIGHT STOMACH CGM KETONES NEGATIVE / TRACE / SMALL / MODERATE / LARGE
DINNER	Total Carbohydrates : ___._ grams	Correction Dose: (BS - ___) / __ (___-___)/__ = (__/__) = ___.__ Carb Dose Calculation: (Meal Carbs / ___) (__._ /___) = ___.__ Correction Dose + Carb Dose Calculation: (_____ + _____) = __.__ OR __ UNITS Correction Dose / Dose Calculation / Rounded to nearest whole number	TIME __ :__ AM / PM LEFT ARM CGM / RIGHT ARM CGM / LEFT LEG CGM / RIGHT LEG CGM / LEFT/RIGHT STOMACH CGM KETONES NEGATIVE / TRACE / SMALL / MODERATE / LARGE
SNACK	Total Carbohydrates : ___._ grams	Carb Dose Calculation: (Meal Carbs / ___) (__._ /___) = ___.__ or __ UNITS NO INSULIN DOSE REQUIRED FOR MEALS/SNACKS UNDER __G OF CARBS OR EQUAL TO __.__ OR LESS	TIME __ :__ AM / PM LEFT ARM CGM / RIGHT ARM CGM / LEFT LEG CGM / RIGHT LEG CGM / LEFT/RIGHT STOMACH CGM KETONES NEGATIVE / TRACE / SMALL / MODERATE / LARGE
BEDTIME __ : __ PM	BLOOD SUGAR ____ UNITS ___ LEFT ARM CGM / RIGHT ARM CGM / LEFT LEG CGM / RIGHT LEG CGM / LEFT/RIGHT STOMACH CGM KETONES NEGATIVE / TRACE / SMALL / MODERATE / LARGE	HYDRATE 2AM BLOOD SUGAR _____ ADDITIONAL BLOOD SUGAR READINGS BS ___ at __ : __ AM/PM BS ___ at __ : __ AM/PM	NOTES MEDICINE

DATE: ______________________________ SUN MON TUES WED THUR FRI SAT

	MEALS AND SNACKS	CARB AND FOOD CALCULATIONS	SHOT DETAILS AND LOCATION
BREAKFAST	Total Carbohydrates : ___._ grams	Correction Dose: (BS - ___) / __ (___-___)/__ = (__/__) = ___.__ Carb Dose Calculation: (Meal Carbs / ___) (__._ /___) = ___.__ Correction Dose + Carb Dose Calculation: (___.__ + ___.__) = __.__ OR __ UNITS Correction Dose / Dose Calculation / Rounded to nearest whole number	TIME __ : __ AM / PM LEFT ARM CGM / RIGHT ARM CGM / LEFT LEG CGM / RIGHT LEG CGM / LEFT/RIGHT STOMACH CGM KETONES NEGATIVE / TRACE / SMALL / MODERATE / LARGE
SNACK	Total Carbohydrates : ___._ grams	Carb Dose Calculation: (Meal Carbs / ___) (__._ /___) = ___.__ or __ UNITS NO INSULIN DOSE REQUIRED FOR MEALS/SNACKS UNDER __G OF CARBS OR EQUAL TO __.__ OR LESS	TIME __ : __ AM / PM LEFT ARM CGM / RIGHT ARM CGM / LEFT LEG CGM / RIGHT LEG CGM / LEFT/RIGHT STOMACH CGM KETONES NEGATIVE / TRACE / SMALL / MODERATE / LARGE
LUNCH	Total Carbohydrates : ___._ grams	Correction Dose: (BS - ___) / __ (___-___)/__ = (__/__) = ___.__ Carb Dose Calculation: (Meal Carbs / ___) (__._ /___) = ___.__ Correction Dose + Carb Dose Calculation: (___.__ + ___.__) = __.__ OR __ UNITS Correction Dose / Dose Calculation / Rounded to nearest whole number	TIME __ : __ AM / PM LEFT ARM CGM / RIGHT ARM CGM / LEFT LEG CGM / RIGHT LEG CGM / LEFT/RIGHT STOMACH CGM KETONES NEGATIVE / TRACE / SMALL / MODERATE / LARGE
SNACK	Total Carbohydrates : ___._ grams	Carb Dose Calculation: (Meal Carbs / ___) (__._ /___) = ___.__ or __ UNITS NO INSULIN DOSE REQUIRED FOR MEALS/SNACKS UNDER __G OF CARBS OR EQUAL TO __.__ OR LESS	TIME __ : __ AM / PM LEFT ARM CGM / RIGHT ARM CGM / LEFT LEG CGM / RIGHT LEG CGM / LEFT/RIGHT STOMACH CGM KETONES NEGATIVE / TRACE / SMALL / MODERATE / LARGE
DINNER	Total Carbohydrates : ___._ grams	Correction Dose: (BS - ___) / __ (___-___)/__ = (__/__) = ___.__ Carb Dose Calculation: (Meal Carbs / ___) (__._ /___) = ___.__ Correction Dose + Carb Dose Calculation: (___.__ + ___.__) = __.__ OR __ UNITS Correction Dose / Dose Calculation / Rounded to nearest whole number	TIME __ : __ AM / PM LEFT ARM CGM / RIGHT ARM CGM / LEFT LEG CGM / RIGHT LEG CGM / LEFT/RIGHT STOMACH CGM KETONES NEGATIVE / TRACE / SMALL / MODERATE / LARGE
SNACK	Total Carbohydrates : ___._ grams	Carb Dose Calculation: (Meal Carbs / ___) (__._ /___) = ___.__ or __ UNITS NO INSULIN DOSE REQUIRED FOR MEALS/SNACKS UNDER __G OF CARBS OR EQUAL TO __.__ OR LESS	TIME __ : __ AM / PM LEFT ARM CGM / RIGHT ARM CGM / LEFT LEG CGM / RIGHT LEG CGM / LEFT/RIGHT STOMACH CGM KETONES NEGATIVE / TRACE / SMALL / MODERATE / LARGE
BEDTIME __ : __ PM	BLOOD SUGAR _____ UNITS ___ LEFT ARM CGM / RIGHT ARM CGM / LEFT LEG CGM / RIGHT LEG CGM / LEFT/RIGHT STOMACH CGM KETONES NEGATIVE / TRACE / SMALL / MODERATE / LARGE	HYDRATE 2AM BLOOD SUGAR _____ ADDITIONAL BLOOD SUGAR READINGS BS ___ at __ : __ AM/PM BS ___ at __ : __ AM/PM	NOTES MEDICINE

DATE: ______________________ SUN MON TUES WED THUR FRI SAT

	MEALS AND SNACKS	CARB AND FOOD CALCULATIONS	SHOT DETAILS AND LOCATION
BREAKFAST	Total Carbohydrates : ___._ grams	Correction Dose: (BS - ___) / __ (___-___)/__ = (__/__) = ___.__ Carb Dose Calculation: (Meal Carbs / ___) (__._ /___) = ___.__ Correction Dose + Carb Dose Calculation: (______ + ______) = __.__ OR __ UNITS Correction Dose Dose Calculation Rounded to nearest whole number	TIME __ : __ AM / PM LEFT ARM CGM / RIGHT ARM CGM / LEFT LEG CGM / RIGHT LEG CGM / LEFT/RIGHT STOMACH CGM KETONES NEGATIVE TRACE SMALL MODERATE LARGE
SNACK	Total Carbohydrates : ___._ grams	Carb Dose Calculation: (Meal Carbs / ___) (__._ /___) = ___.__ or __ UNITS NO INSULIN DOSE REQUIRED FOR MEALS/SNACKS UNDER __G OF CARBS OR EQUAL TO __.__ OR LESS	TIME __ : __ AM / PM LEFT ARM CGM / RIGHT ARM CGM / LEFT LEG CGM / RIGHT LEG CGM / LEFT/RIGHT STOMACH CGM KETONES NEGATIVE TRACE SMALL MODERATE LARGE
LUNCH	Total Carbohydrates : ___._ grams	Correction Dose: (BS - ___) / __ (___-___)/__ = (__/__) = ___.__ Carb Dose Calculation: (Meal Carbs / ___) (__._ /___) = ___.__ Correction Dose + Carb Dose Calculation: (______ + ______) = __.__ OR __ UNITS Correction Dose Dose Calculation Rounded to nearest whole number	TIME __ : __ AM / PM LEFT ARM CGM / RIGHT ARM CGM / LEFT LEG CGM / RIGHT LEG CGM / LEFT/RIGHT STOMACH CGM KETONES NEGATIVE TRACE SMALL MODERATE LARGE
SNACK	Total Carbohydrates : ___._ grams	Carb Dose Calculation: (Meal Carbs / ___) (__._ /___) = ___.__ or __ UNITS NO INSULIN DOSE REQUIRED FOR MEALS/SNACKS UNDER __G OF CARBS OR EQUAL TO __.__ OR LESS	TIME __ : __ AM / PM LEFT ARM CGM / RIGHT ARM CGM / LEFT LEG CGM / RIGHT LEG CGM / LEFT/RIGHT STOMACH CGM KETONES NEGATIVE TRACE SMALL MODERATE LARGE
DINNER	Total Carbohydrates : ___._ grams	Correction Dose: (BS - ___) / __ (___-___)/__ = (__/__) = ___.__ Carb Dose Calculation: (Meal Carbs / ___) (__._ /___) = ___.__ Correction Dose + Carb Dose Calculation: (______ + ______) = __.__ OR __ UNITS Correction Dose Dose Calculation Rounded to nearest whole number	TIME __ : __ AM / PM LEFT ARM CGM / RIGHT ARM CGM / LEFT LEG CGM / RIGHT LEG CGM / LEFT/RIGHT STOMACH CGM KETONES NEGATIVE TRACE SMALL MODERATE LARGE
SNACK	Total Carbohydrates : ___._ grams	Carb Dose Calculation: (Meal Carbs / ___) (__._ /___) = ___.__ or __ UNITS NO INSULIN DOSE REQUIRED FOR MEALS/SNACKS UNDER __G OF CARBS OR EQUAL TO __.__ OR LESS	TIME __ : __ AM / PM LEFT ARM CGM / RIGHT ARM CGM / LEFT LEG CGM / RIGHT LEG CGM / LEFT/RIGHT STOMACH CGM KETONES NEGATIVE TRACE SMALL MODERATE LARGE
BEDTIME __ : __ PM	BLOOD SUGAR ____ UNITS ___ LEFT ARM CGM / RIGHT ARM CGM / LEFT LEG CGM / RIGHT LEG CGM / LEFT/RIGHT STOMACH CGM KETONES NEGATIVE TRACE SMALL MODERATE LARGE	HYDRATE 2AM BLOOD SUGAR ____ ADDITIONAL BLOOD SUGAR READINGS BS ___ at __ : __ AM/PM BS ___ at __ : __ AM/PM	NOTES MEDICINE

DATE: ______________________ SUN MON TUES WED THUR FRI SAT

	MEALS AND SNACKS	CARB AND FOOD CALCULATIONS	SHOT DETAILS AND LOCATION
BREAKFAST	Total Carbohydrates : ___._ grams	Correction Dose: (BS - ___) / __ (___-___)/__ = (__/__) = ___.__ Carb Dose Calculation: (Meal Carbs / ___) (__._ /___) = ___.__ Correction Dose + Carb Dose Calculation: (___.__ + ___.__) = __.__ OR __ UNITS Correction Dose Dose Calculation Rounded to nearest whole number	TIME __ : __ AM / PM LEFT ARM CGM, RIGHT ARM CGM, LEFT LEG CGM, RIGHT LEG CGM, LEFT/RIGHT STOMACH CGM KETONES NEGATIVE TRACE SMALL MODERATE LARGE
SNACK	Total Carbohydrates : ___._ grams	Carb Dose Calculation: (Meal Carbs / ___) (__._ /___) = ___.__ or __ UNITS NO INSULIN DOSE REQUIRED FOR MEALS/SNACKS UNDER __G OF CARBS OR EQUAL TO __.__ OR LESS	TIME __ : __ AM / PM LEFT ARM CGM, RIGHT ARM CGM, LEFT LEG CGM, RIGHT LEG CGM, LEFT/RIGHT STOMACH CGM KETONES NEGATIVE TRACE SMALL MODERATE LARGE
LUNCH	Total Carbohydrates : ___._ grams	Correction Dose: (BS - ___) / __ (___-___)/__ = (__/__) = ___.__ Carb Dose Calculation: (Meal Carbs / ___) (__._ /___) = ___.__ Correction Dose + Carb Dose Calculation: (___.__ + ___.__) = __.__ OR __ UNITS Correction Dose Dose Calculation Rounded to nearest whole number	TIME __ : __ AM / PM LEFT ARM CGM, RIGHT ARM CGM, LEFT LEG CGM, RIGHT LEG CGM, LEFT/RIGHT STOMACH CGM KETONES NEGATIVE TRACE SMALL MODERATE LARGE
SNACK	Total Carbohydrates : ___._ grams	Carb Dose Calculation: (Meal Carbs / ___) (__._ /___) = ___.__ or __ UNITS NO INSULIN DOSE REQUIRED FOR MEALS/SNACKS UNDER __G OF CARBS OR EQUAL TO __.__ OR LESS	TIME __ : __ AM / PM LEFT ARM CGM, RIGHT ARM CGM, LEFT LEG CGM, RIGHT LEG CGM, LEFT/RIGHT STOMACH CGM KETONES NEGATIVE TRACE SMALL MODERATE LARGE
DINNER	Total Carbohydrates : ___._ grams	Correction Dose: (BS - ___) / __ (___-___)/__ = (__/__) = ___.__ Carb Dose Calculation: (Meal Carbs / ___) (__._ /___) = ___.__ Correction Dose + Carb Dose Calculation: (___.__ + ___.__) = __.__ OR __ UNITS Correction Dose Dose Calculation Rounded to nearest whole number	TIME __ : __ AM / PM LEFT ARM CGM, RIGHT ARM CGM, LEFT LEG CGM, RIGHT LEG CGM, LEFT/RIGHT STOMACH CGM KETONES NEGATIVE TRACE SMALL MODERATE LARGE
SNACK	Total Carbohydrates : ___._ grams	Carb Dose Calculation: (Meal Carbs / ___) (__._ /___) = ___.__ or __ UNITS NO INSULIN DOSE REQUIRED FOR MEALS/SNACKS UNDER __G OF CARBS OR EQUAL TO __.__ OR LESS	TIME __ : __ AM / PM LEFT ARM CGM, RIGHT ARM CGM, LEFT LEG CGM, RIGHT LEG CGM, LEFT/RIGHT STOMACH CGM KETONES NEGATIVE TRACE SMALL MODERATE LARGE
BEDTIME __ : __ PM	BLOOD SUGAR _____ UNITS ___ LEFT ARM CGM, RIGHT ARM CGM, LEFT LEG CGM, RIGHT LEG CGM, LEFT/RIGHT STOMACH CGM KETONES NEGATIVE TRACE SMALL MODERATE LARGE	HYDRATE 2AM BLOOD SUGAR _____ ADDITIONAL BLOOD SUGAR READINGS BS ___ at __ : __ AM/PM BS ___ at __ : __ AM/PM	NOTES MEDICINE

DATE: ____________________ SUN MON TUES WED THUR FRI SAT

	MEALS AND SNACKS	CARB AND FOOD CALCULATIONS	SHOT DETAILS AND LOCATION
BREAKFAST	Total Carbohydrates : ___._ grams	Correction Dose: (BS - ___) / __ (___-___)/__ = (__/__) = ___.__ Carb Dose Calculation: (Meal Carbs / ___) (__._ /___) = ___.__ Correction Dose + Carb Dose Calculation: (_____ + _____) = __.__ OR __ UNITS Correction Dose, Dose Calculation, Rounded to nearest whole number	TIME __ :__ AM / PM LEFT ARM CGM / RIGHT ARM CGM / LEFT LEG CGM / RIGHT LEG CGM / LEFT/RIGHT STOMACH CGM KETONES NEGATIVE TRACE SMALL MODERATE LARGE
SNACK	Total Carbohydrates : ___._ grams	Carb Dose Calculation: (Meal Carbs / ___) (__._ /___) = ___.__ or __ UNITS NO INSULIN DOSE REQUIRED FOR MEALS/SNACKS UNDER __G OF CARBS OR EQUAL TO __.__ OR LESS	TIME __ :__ AM / PM LEFT ARM CGM / RIGHT ARM CGM / LEFT LEG CGM / RIGHT LEG CGM / LEFT/RIGHT STOMACH CGM KETONES NEGATIVE TRACE SMALL MODERATE LARGE
LUNCH	Total Carbohydrates : ___._ grams	Correction Dose: (BS - ___) / __ (___-___)/__ = (__/__) = ___.__ Carb Dose Calculation: (Meal Carbs / ___) (__._ /___) = ___.__ Correction Dose + Carb Dose Calculation: (_____ + _____) = __.__ OR __ UNITS Correction Dose, Dose Calculation, Rounded to nearest whole number	TIME __ :__ AM / PM LEFT ARM CGM / RIGHT ARM CGM / LEFT LEG CGM / RIGHT LEG CGM / LEFT/RIGHT STOMACH CGM KETONES NEGATIVE TRACE SMALL MODERATE LARGE
SNACK	Total Carbohydrates : ___._ grams	Carb Dose Calculation: (Meal Carbs / ___) (__._ /___) = ___.__ or __ UNITS NO INSULIN DOSE REQUIRED FOR MEALS/SNACKS UNDER __G OF CARBS OR EQUAL TO __.__ OR LESS	TIME __ :__ AM / PM LEFT ARM CGM / RIGHT ARM CGM / LEFT LEG CGM / RIGHT LEG CGM / LEFT/RIGHT STOMACH CGM KETONES NEGATIVE TRACE SMALL MODERATE LARGE
DINNER	Total Carbohydrates : ___._ grams	Correction Dose: (BS - ___) / __ (___-___)/__ = (__/__) = ___.__ Carb Dose Calculation: (Meal Carbs / ___) (__._ /___) = ___.__ Correction Dose + Carb Dose Calculation: (_____ + _____) = __.__ OR __ UNITS Correction Dose, Dose Calculation, Rounded to nearest whole number	TIME __ :__ AM / PM LEFT ARM CGM / RIGHT ARM CGM / LEFT LEG CGM / RIGHT LEG CGM / LEFT/RIGHT STOMACH CGM KETONES NEGATIVE TRACE SMALL MODERATE LARGE
SNACK	Total Carbohydrates : ___._ grams	Carb Dose Calculation: (Meal Carbs / ___) (__._ /___) = ___.__ or __ UNITS NO INSULIN DOSE REQUIRED FOR MEALS/SNACKS UNDER __G OF CARBS OR EQUAL TO __.__ OR LESS	TIME __ :__ AM / PM LEFT ARM CGM / RIGHT ARM CGM / LEFT LEG CGM / RIGHT LEG CGM / LEFT/RIGHT STOMACH CGM KETONES NEGATIVE TRACE SMALL MODERATE LARGE
BEDTIME __ : __ PM	BLOOD SUGAR _____ UNITS ___ LEFT ARM CGM / RIGHT ARM CGM / LEFT LEG CGM / RIGHT LEG CGM / LEFT/RIGHT STOMACH CGM KETONES NEGATIVE TRACE SMALL MODERATE LARGE	HYDRATE 2AM BLOOD SUGAR _____ ADDITIONAL BLOOD SUGAR READINGS BS ___ at __ : __ AM/PM BS ___ at __ : __ AM/PM	NOTES MEDICINE

DATE: ______________________ SUN MON TUES WED THUR FRI SAT

	MEALS AND SNACKS	CARB AND FOOD CALCULATIONS	SHOT DETAILS AND LOCATION
BREAKFAST	Total Carbohydrates : ___._ grams	Correction Dose: (BS - ___) / __ (___-___)/__ = (__/__) = ___.__ Carb Dose Calculation: (Meal Carbs / ___) (__._ /___) = ___.__ Correction Dose + Carb Dose Calculation: (___.__ + ___.__) = __.__ OR __ UNITS Correction Dose / Dose Calculation / Rounded to nearest whole number	TIME __ : __ AM / PM LEFT ARM CGM / RIGHT ARM CGM / LEFT LEG CGM / RIGHT LEG CGM / LEFT/RIGHT STOMACH CGM KETONES NEGATIVE / TRACE / SMALL / MODERATE / LARGE
SNACK	Total Carbohydrates : ___._ grams	Carb Dose Calculation: (Meal Carbs / ___) (__._ /___) = ___.__ or __ UNITS NO INSULIN DOSE REQUIRED FOR MEALS/SNACKS UNDER __G OF CARBS OR EQUAL TO __.__ OR LESS	TIME __ : __ AM / PM LEFT ARM CGM / RIGHT ARM CGM / LEFT LEG CGM / RIGHT LEG CGM / LEFT/RIGHT STOMACH CGM KETONES NEGATIVE / TRACE / SMALL / MODERATE / LARGE
LUNCH	Total Carbohydrates : ___._ grams	Correction Dose: (BS - ___) / __ (___-___)/__ = (__/__) = ___.__ Carb Dose Calculation: (Meal Carbs / ___) (__._ /___) = ___.__ Correction Dose + Carb Dose Calculation: (___.__ + ___.__) = __.__ OR __ UNITS Correction Dose / Dose Calculation / Rounded to nearest whole number	TIME __ : __ AM / PM LEFT ARM CGM / RIGHT ARM CGM / LEFT LEG CGM / RIGHT LEG CGM / LEFT/RIGHT STOMACH CGM KETONES NEGATIVE / TRACE / SMALL / MODERATE / LARGE
SNACK	Total Carbohydrates : ___._ grams	Carb Dose Calculation: (Meal Carbs / ___) (__._ /___) = ___.__ or __ UNITS NO INSULIN DOSE REQUIRED FOR MEALS/SNACKS UNDER __G OF CARBS OR EQUAL TO __.__ OR LESS	TIME __ : __ AM / PM LEFT ARM CGM / RIGHT ARM CGM / LEFT LEG CGM / RIGHT LEG CGM / LEFT/RIGHT STOMACH CGM KETONES NEGATIVE / TRACE / SMALL / MODERATE / LARGE
DINNER	Total Carbohydrates : ___._ grams	Correction Dose: (BS - ___) / __ (___-___)/__ = (__/__) = ___.__ Carb Dose Calculation: (Meal Carbs / ___) (__._ /___) = ___.__ Correction Dose + Carb Dose Calculation: (___.__ + ___.__) = __.__ OR __ UNITS Correction Dose / Dose Calculation / Rounded to nearest whole number	TIME __ : __ AM / PM LEFT ARM CGM / RIGHT ARM CGM / LEFT LEG CGM / RIGHT LEG CGM / LEFT/RIGHT STOMACH CGM KETONES NEGATIVE / TRACE / SMALL / MODERATE / LARGE
SNACK	Total Carbohydrates : ___._ grams	Carb Dose Calculation: (Meal Carbs / ___) (__._ /___) = ___.__ or __ UNITS NO INSULIN DOSE REQUIRED FOR MEALS/SNACKS UNDER __G OF CARBS OR EQUAL TO __.__ OR LESS	TIME __ : __ AM / PM LEFT ARM CGM / RIGHT ARM CGM / LEFT LEG CGM / RIGHT LEG CGM / LEFT/RIGHT STOMACH CGM KETONES NEGATIVE / TRACE / SMALL / MODERATE / LARGE
BEDTIME __ : __ PM	BLOOD SUGAR ____ UNITS ___ LEFT ARM CGM / RIGHT ARM CGM / LEFT LEG CGM / RIGHT LEG CGM / LEFT/RIGHT STOMACH CGM KETONES NEGATIVE / TRACE / SMALL / MODERATE / LARGE	HYDRATE 2AM BLOOD SUGAR ____ ADDITIONAL BLOOD SUGAR READINGS BS ___ at __ : __ AM/PM BS ___ at __ : __ AM/PM	NOTES MEDICINE

DATE: ______________________ SUN MON TUES WED THUR FRI SAT

	MEALS AND SNACKS	CARB AND FOOD CALCULATIONS	SHOT DETAILS AND LOCATION
BREAKFAST	Total Carbohydrates : ___._ grams	Correction Dose: (BS - ___) / __ (___-___)/__ = (__/__) = ___.__ Carb Dose Calculation: (Meal Carbs / ___) (__._ /___) = ___.__ Correction Dose + Carb Dose Calculation: (_____ + _____) = __.__ OR __ UNITS Correction Dose · Dose Calculation · Rounded to nearest whole number	TIME __ : __ AM / PM LEFT ARM CGM · RIGHT ARM CGM · LEFT LEG CGM · RIGHT LEG CGM · LEFT/RIGHT STOMACH CGM KETONES NEGATIVE · TRACE · SMALL · MODERATE · LARGE
SNACK	Total Carbohydrates : ___._ grams	Carb Dose Calculation: (Meal Carbs / ___) (__._ /___) = ___.__ or __ UNITS NO INSULIN DOSE REQUIRED FOR MEALS/SNACKS UNDER __G OF CARBS OR EQUAL TO __.__ OR LESS	TIME __ : __ AM / PM LEFT ARM CGM · RIGHT ARM CGM · LEFT LEG CGM · RIGHT LEG CGM · LEFT/RIGHT STOMACH CGM KETONES NEGATIVE · TRACE · SMALL · MODERATE · LARGE
LUNCH	Total Carbohydrates : ___._ grams	Correction Dose: (BS - ___) / __ (___-___)/__ = (__/__) = ___.__ Carb Dose Calculation: (Meal Carbs / ___) (__._ /___) = ___.__ Correction Dose + Carb Dose Calculation: (_____ + _____) = __.__ OR __ UNITS Correction Dose · Dose Calculation · Rounded to nearest whole number	TIME __ : __ AM / PM LEFT ARM CGM · RIGHT ARM CGM · LEFT LEG CGM · RIGHT LEG CGM · LEFT/RIGHT STOMACH CGM KETONES NEGATIVE · TRACE · SMALL · MODERATE · LARGE
SNACK	Total Carbohydrates : ___._ grams	Carb Dose Calculation: (Meal Carbs / ___) (__._ /___) = ___.__ or __ UNITS NO INSULIN DOSE REQUIRED FOR MEALS/SNACKS UNDER __G OF CARBS OR EQUAL TO __.__ OR LESS	TIME __ : __ AM / PM LEFT ARM CGM · RIGHT ARM CGM · LEFT LEG CGM · RIGHT LEG CGM · LEFT/RIGHT STOMACH CGM KETONES NEGATIVE · TRACE · SMALL · MODERATE · LARGE
DINNER	Total Carbohydrates : ___._ grams	Correction Dose: (BS - ___) / __ (___-___)/__ = (__/__) = ___.__ Carb Dose Calculation: (Meal Carbs / ___) (__._ /___) = ___.__ Correction Dose + Carb Dose Calculation: (_____ + _____) = __.__ OR __ UNITS Correction Dose · Dose Calculation · Rounded to nearest whole number	TIME __ : __ AM / PM LEFT ARM CGM · RIGHT ARM CGM · LEFT LEG CGM · RIGHT LEG CGM · LEFT/RIGHT STOMACH CGM KETONES NEGATIVE · TRACE · SMALL · MODERATE · LARGE
SNACK	Total Carbohydrates : ___._ grams	Carb Dose Calculation: (Meal Carbs / ___) (__._ /___) = ___.__ or __ UNITS NO INSULIN DOSE REQUIRED FOR MEALS/SNACKS UNDER __G OF CARBS OR EQUAL TO __.__ OR LESS	TIME __ : __ AM / PM LEFT ARM CGM · RIGHT ARM CGM · LEFT LEG CGM · RIGHT LEG CGM · LEFT/RIGHT STOMACH CGM KETONES NEGATIVE · TRACE · SMALL · MODERATE · LARGE
BEDTIME __ : __ PM	BLOOD SUGAR ____ · UNITS ___ LEFT ARM CGM · RIGHT ARM CGM · LEFT LEG CGM · RIGHT LEG CGM · LEFT/RIGHT STOMACH CGM KETONES NEGATIVE · TRACE · SMALL · MODERATE · LARGE	HYDRATE 2AM BLOOD SUGAR ____ ADDITIONAL BLOOD SUGAR READINGS BS ___ at __ : __ AM/PM BS ___ at __ : __ AM/PM	NOTES MEDICINE

DATE: ______________________ SUN MON TUES WED THUR FRI SAT

	MEALS AND SNACKS	CARB AND FOOD CALCULATIONS	SHOT DETAILS AND LOCATION
BREAKFAST	Total Carbohydrates : ___.__ grams	Correction Dose: (BS - ___) / __ (___-___)/__ = (__/__) = ___.__ Carb Dose Calculation: (Meal Carbs / ___) (__.__ /___) = ___.__ Correction Dose + Carb Dose Calculation: (_____ + _____) = __.__ OR __ UNITS Correction Dose · Dose Calculation · Rounded to nearest whole number	TIME __ : __ AM / PM LEFT ARM CGM · RIGHT ARM CGM · LEFT LEG CGM · RIGHT LEG CGM · LEFT/RIGHT STOMACH CGM KETONES NEGATIVE · TRACE · SMALL · MODERATE · LARGE
SNACK	Total Carbohydrates : ___.__ grams	Carb Dose Calculation: (Meal Carbs / ___) (__.__ /___) = ___.__ or __ UNITS NO INSULIN DOSE REQUIRED FOR MEALS/SNACKS UNDER __G OF CARBS OR EQUAL TO __.__ OR LESS	TIME __ : __ AM / PM LEFT ARM CGM · RIGHT ARM CGM · LEFT LEG CGM · RIGHT LEG CGM · LEFT/RIGHT STOMACH CGM KETONES NEGATIVE · TRACE · SMALL · MODERATE · LARGE
LUNCH	Total Carbohydrates : ___.__ grams	Correction Dose: (BS - ___) / __ (___-___)/__ = (__/__) = ___.__ Carb Dose Calculation: (Meal Carbs / ___) (__.__ /___) = ___.__ Correction Dose + Carb Dose Calculation: (_____ + _____) = __.__ OR __ UNITS Correction Dose · Dose Calculation · Rounded to nearest whole number	TIME __ : __ AM / PM LEFT ARM CGM · RIGHT ARM CGM · LEFT LEG CGM · RIGHT LEG CGM · LEFT/RIGHT STOMACH CGM KETONES NEGATIVE · TRACE · SMALL · MODERATE · LARGE
SNACK	Total Carbohydrates : ___.__ grams	Carb Dose Calculation: (Meal Carbs / ___) (__.__ /___) = ___.__ or __ UNITS NO INSULIN DOSE REQUIRED FOR MEALS/SNACKS UNDER __G OF CARBS OR EQUAL TO __.__ OR LESS	TIME __ : __ AM / PM LEFT ARM CGM · RIGHT ARM CGM · LEFT LEG CGM · RIGHT LEG CGM · LEFT/RIGHT STOMACH CGM KETONES NEGATIVE · TRACE · SMALL · MODERATE · LARGE
DINNER	Total Carbohydrates : ___.__ grams	Correction Dose: (BS - ___) / __ (___-___)/__ = (__/__) = ___.__ Carb Dose Calculation: (Meal Carbs / ___) (__.__ /___) = ___.__ Correction Dose + Carb Dose Calculation: (_____ + _____) = __.__ OR __ UNITS Correction Dose · Dose Calculation · Rounded to nearest whole number	TIME __ : __ AM / PM LEFT ARM CGM · RIGHT ARM CGM · LEFT LEG CGM · RIGHT LEG CGM · LEFT/RIGHT STOMACH CGM KETONES NEGATIVE · TRACE · SMALL · MODERATE · LARGE
SNACK	Total Carbohydrates : ___.__ grams	Carb Dose Calculation: (Meal Carbs / ___) (__.__ /___) = ___.__ or __ UNITS NO INSULIN DOSE REQUIRED FOR MEALS/SNACKS UNDER __G OF CARBS OR EQUAL TO __.__ OR LESS	TIME __ : __ AM / PM LEFT ARM CGM · RIGHT ARM CGM · LEFT LEG CGM · RIGHT LEG CGM · LEFT/RIGHT STOMACH CGM KETONES NEGATIVE · TRACE · SMALL · MODERATE · LARGE
BEDTIME __ : __ PM	BLOOD SUGAR _____ UNITS ___ LEFT ARM CGM · RIGHT ARM CGM · LEFT LEG CGM · RIGHT LEG CGM · LEFT/RIGHT STOMACH CGM KETONES NEGATIVE · TRACE · SMALL · MODERATE · LARGE	HYDRATE 2AM BLOOD SUGAR _____ ADDITIONAL BLOOD SUGAR READINGS BS ___ at __ : __ AM/PM BS ___ at __ : __ AM/PM	NOTES MEDICINE

DATE: ______________________ SUN MON TUES WED THUR FRI SAT

	MEALS AND SNACKS	CARB AND FOOD CALCULATIONS	SHOT DETAILS AND LOCATION
BREAKFAST	Total Carbohydrates : ___._ grams	Correction Dose: (BS - ___) / __ (___-___)/__ = (__/__) = ___.__ Carb Dose Calculation: (Meal Carbs / ___) (__._ /___) = ___.__ Correction Dose + Carb Dose Calculation: (_____ + _____) = __.__ OR __ UNITS Correction Dose Dose Calculation Rounded to nearest whole number	TIME __ :__ AM / PM LEFT ARM CGM / RIGHT ARM CGM / LEFT LEG CGM / RIGHT LEG CGM / LEFT/RIGHT STOMACH CGM KETONES NEGATIVE TRACE SMALL MODERATE LARGE
SNACK	Total Carbohydrates : ___._ grams	Carb Dose Calculation: (Meal Carbs / ___) (__._ /___) = ___.__ or __ UNITS NO INSULIN DOSE REQUIRED FOR MEALS/SNACKS UNDER __G OF CARBS OR EQUAL TO __.__ OR LESS	TIME __ :__ AM / PM LEFT ARM CGM / RIGHT ARM CGM / LEFT LEG CGM / RIGHT LEG CGM / LEFT/RIGHT STOMACH CGM KETONES NEGATIVE TRACE SMALL MODERATE LARGE
LUNCH	Total Carbohydrates : ___._ grams	Correction Dose: (BS - ___) / __ (___-___)/__ = (__/__) = ___.__ Carb Dose Calculation: (Meal Carbs / ___) (__._ /___) = ___.__ Correction Dose + Carb Dose Calculation: (_____ + _____) = __.__ OR __ UNITS Correction Dose Dose Calculation Rounded to nearest whole number	TIME __ :__ AM / PM LEFT ARM CGM / RIGHT ARM CGM / LEFT LEG CGM / RIGHT LEG CGM / LEFT/RIGHT STOMACH CGM KETONES NEGATIVE TRACE SMALL MODERATE LARGE
SNACK	Total Carbohydrates : ___._ grams	Carb Dose Calculation: (Meal Carbs / ___) (__._ /___) = ___.__ or __ UNITS NO INSULIN DOSE REQUIRED FOR MEALS/SNACKS UNDER __G OF CARBS OR EQUAL TO __.__ OR LESS	TIME __ :__ AM / PM LEFT ARM CGM / RIGHT ARM CGM / LEFT LEG CGM / RIGHT LEG CGM / LEFT/RIGHT STOMACH CGM KETONES NEGATIVE TRACE SMALL MODERATE LARGE
DINNER	Total Carbohydrates : ___._ grams	Correction Dose: (BS - ___) / __ (___-___)/__ = (__/__) = ___.__ Carb Dose Calculation: (Meal Carbs / ___) (__._ /___) = ___.__ Correction Dose + Carb Dose Calculation: (_____ + _____) = __.__ OR __ UNITS Correction Dose Dose Calculation Rounded to nearest whole number	TIME __ :__ AM / PM LEFT ARM CGM / RIGHT ARM CGM / LEFT LEG CGM / RIGHT LEG CGM / LEFT/RIGHT STOMACH CGM KETONES NEGATIVE TRACE SMALL MODERATE LARGE
SNACK	Total Carbohydrates : ___._ grams	Carb Dose Calculation: (Meal Carbs / ___) (__._ /___) = ___.__ or __ UNITS NO INSULIN DOSE REQUIRED FOR MEALS/SNACKS UNDER __G OF CARBS OR EQUAL TO __.__ OR LESS	TIME __ :__ AM / PM LEFT ARM CGM / RIGHT ARM CGM / LEFT LEG CGM / RIGHT LEG CGM / LEFT/RIGHT STOMACH CGM KETONES NEGATIVE TRACE SMALL MODERATE LARGE
BEDTIME __ : __ PM	BLOOD SUGAR ____ UNITS ___ LEFT ARM CGM / RIGHT ARM CGM / LEFT LEG CGM / RIGHT LEG CGM / LEFT/RIGHT STOMACH CGM KETONES NEGATIVE TRACE SMALL MODERATE LARGE	HYDRATE 2AM BLOOD SUGAR ____ ADDITIONAL BLOOD SUGAR READINGS BS ___ at __ : __ AM/PM BS ___ at __ : __ AM/PM	NOTES MEDICINE

DATE: ______________________ SUN MON TUES WED THUR FRI SAT

	MEALS AND SNACKS	CARB AND FOOD CALCULATIONS	SHOT DETAILS AND LOCATION
BREAKFAST	Total Carbohydrates : ___._ grams	Correction Dose: (BS - ___) / __ (___-___)/__ = (__/__) = ___.__ Carb Dose Calculation: (Meal Carbs / ___) (__._ /___) = ___.__ Correction Dose + Carb Dose Calculation: (___.__ + ___.__) = __.__ OR __ UNITS Correction Dose Dose Calculation Rounded to nearest whole number	TIME __ : __ AM / PM LEFT ARM CGM, RIGHT ARM CGM, LEFT LEG CGM, RIGHT LEG CGM, LEFT/RIGHT STOMACH CGM KETONES NEGATIVE TRACE SMALL MODERATE LARGE
SNACK	Total Carbohydrates : ___._ grams	Carb Dose Calculation: (Meal Carbs / ___) (__._ /___) = ___.__ or __ UNITS NO INSULIN DOSE REQUIRED FOR MEALS/SNACKS UNDER __G OF CARBS OR EQUAL TO __.__ OR LESS	TIME __ : __ AM / PM LEFT ARM CGM, RIGHT ARM CGM, LEFT LEG CGM, RIGHT LEG CGM, LEFT/RIGHT STOMACH CGM KETONES NEGATIVE TRACE SMALL MODERATE LARGE
LUNCH	Total Carbohydrates : ___._ grams	Correction Dose: (BS - ___) / __ (___-___)/__ = (__/__) = ___.__ Carb Dose Calculation: (Meal Carbs / ___) (__._ /___) = ___.__ Correction Dose + Carb Dose Calculation: (___.__ + ___.__) = __.__ OR __ UNITS Correction Dose Dose Calculation Rounded to nearest whole number	TIME __ : __ AM / PM LEFT ARM CGM, RIGHT ARM CGM, LEFT LEG CGM, RIGHT LEG CGM, LEFT/RIGHT STOMACH CGM KETONES NEGATIVE TRACE SMALL MODERATE LARGE
SNACK	Total Carbohydrates : ___._ grams	Carb Dose Calculation: (Meal Carbs / ___) (__._ /___) = ___.__ or __ UNITS NO INSULIN DOSE REQUIRED FOR MEALS/SNACKS UNDER __G OF CARBS OR EQUAL TO __.__ OR LESS	TIME __ : __ AM / PM LEFT ARM CGM, RIGHT ARM CGM, LEFT LEG CGM, RIGHT LEG CGM, LEFT/RIGHT STOMACH CGM KETONES NEGATIVE TRACE SMALL MODERATE LARGE
DINNER	Total Carbohydrates : ___._ grams	Correction Dose: (BS - ___) / __ (___-___)/__ = (__/__) = ___.__ Carb Dose Calculation: (Meal Carbs / ___) (__._ /___) = ___.__ Correction Dose + Carb Dose Calculation: (___.__ + ___.__) = __.__ OR __ UNITS Correction Dose Dose Calculation Rounded to nearest whole number	TIME __ : __ AM / PM LEFT ARM CGM, RIGHT ARM CGM, LEFT LEG CGM, RIGHT LEG CGM, LEFT/RIGHT STOMACH CGM KETONES NEGATIVE TRACE SMALL MODERATE LARGE
SNACK	Total Carbohydrates : ___._ grams	Carb Dose Calculation: (Meal Carbs / ___) (__._ /___) = ___.__ or __ UNITS NO INSULIN DOSE REQUIRED FOR MEALS/SNACKS UNDER __G OF CARBS OR EQUAL TO __.__ OR LESS	TIME __ : __ AM / PM LEFT ARM CGM, RIGHT ARM CGM, LEFT LEG CGM, RIGHT LEG CGM, LEFT/RIGHT STOMACH CGM KETONES NEGATIVE TRACE SMALL MODERATE LARGE
BEDTIME __ : __ PM	BLOOD SUGAR _____ UNITS ___ LEFT ARM CGM, RIGHT ARM CGM, LEFT LEG CGM, RIGHT LEG CGM, LEFT/RIGHT STOMACH CGM KETONES NEGATIVE TRACE SMALL MODERATE LARGE	HYDRATE 2AM BLOOD SUGAR _____ ADDITIONAL BLOOD SUGAR READINGS BS ___ at __ : __ AM/PM BS ___ at __ : __ AM/PM	NOTES MEDICINE

DATE: ______________________ SUN MON TUES WED THUR FRI SAT

	MEALS AND SNACKS	CARB AND FOOD CALCULATIONS	SHOT DETAILS AND LOCATION
BREAKFAST	Total Carbohydrates : ___._ grams	Correction Dose: (BS - ___) / __ (___-___)/__ = (__/__) = ___.__ Carb Dose Calculation: (Meal Carbs / ___) (__._ /___) = ___.__ Correction Dose + Carb Dose Calculation: (______ + ______) = __.__ OR __ UNITS Correction Dose / Dose Calculation / Rounded to nearest whole number	TIME __ : __ AM / PM LEFT ARM CGM / RIGHT ARM CGM / LEFT LEG CGM / RIGHT LEG CGM / LEFT/RIGHT STOMACH CGM KETONES NEGATIVE / TRACE / SMALL / MODERATE / LARGE
SNACK	Total Carbohydrates : ___._ grams	Carb Dose Calculation: (Meal Carbs / ___) (__._ /___) = ___.__ or __ UNITS NO INSULIN DOSE REQUIRED FOR MEALS/SNACKS UNDER __G OF CARBS OR EQUAL TO __.__ OR LESS	TIME __ : __ AM / PM LEFT ARM CGM / RIGHT ARM CGM / LEFT LEG CGM / RIGHT LEG CGM / LEFT/RIGHT STOMACH CGM KETONES NEGATIVE / TRACE / SMALL / MODERATE / LARGE
LUNCH	Total Carbohydrates : ___._ grams	Correction Dose: (BS - ___) / __ (___-___)/__ = (__/__) = ___.__ Carb Dose Calculation: (Meal Carbs / ___) (__._ /___) = ___.__ Correction Dose + Carb Dose Calculation: (______ + ______) = __.__ OR __ UNITS Correction Dose / Dose Calculation / Rounded to nearest whole number	TIME __ : __ AM / PM LEFT ARM CGM / RIGHT ARM CGM / LEFT LEG CGM / RIGHT LEG CGM / LEFT/RIGHT STOMACH CGM KETONES NEGATIVE / TRACE / SMALL / MODERATE / LARGE
SNACK	Total Carbohydrates : ___._ grams	Carb Dose Calculation: (Meal Carbs / ___) (__._ /___) = ___.__ or __ UNITS NO INSULIN DOSE REQUIRED FOR MEALS/SNACKS UNDER __G OF CARBS OR EQUAL TO __.__ OR LESS	TIME __ : __ AM / PM LEFT ARM CGM / RIGHT ARM CGM / LEFT LEG CGM / RIGHT LEG CGM / LEFT/RIGHT STOMACH CGM KETONES NEGATIVE / TRACE / SMALL / MODERATE / LARGE
DINNER	Total Carbohydrates : ___._ grams	Correction Dose: (BS - ___) / __ (___-___)/__ = (__/__) = ___.__ Carb Dose Calculation: (Meal Carbs / ___) (__._ /___) = ___.__ Correction Dose + Carb Dose Calculation: (______ + ______) = __.__ OR __ UNITS Correction Dose / Dose Calculation / Rounded to nearest whole number	TIME __ : __ AM / PM LEFT ARM CGM / RIGHT ARM CGM / LEFT LEG CGM / RIGHT LEG CGM / LEFT/RIGHT STOMACH CGM KETONES NEGATIVE / TRACE / SMALL / MODERATE / LARGE
SNACK	Total Carbohydrates : ___._ grams	Carb Dose Calculation: (Meal Carbs / ___) (__._ /___) = ___.__ or __ UNITS NO INSULIN DOSE REQUIRED FOR MEALS/SNACKS UNDER __G OF CARBS OR EQUAL TO __.__ OR LESS	TIME __ : __ AM / PM LEFT ARM CGM / RIGHT ARM CGM / LEFT LEG CGM / RIGHT LEG CGM / LEFT/RIGHT STOMACH CGM KETONES NEGATIVE / TRACE / SMALL / MODERATE / LARGE
BEDTIME __ : __ PM	BLOOD SUGAR _____ UNITS ___ LEFT ARM CGM / RIGHT ARM CGM / LEFT LEG CGM / RIGHT LEG CGM / LEFT/RIGHT STOMACH CGM KETONES NEGATIVE / TRACE / SMALL / MODERATE / LARGE	HYDRATE 2AM BLOOD SUGAR _____ ADDITIONAL BLOOD SUGAR READINGS BS ___ at __ : __ AM/PM BS ___ at __ : __ AM/PM	NOTES MEDICINE

DATE: ______________________ SUN MON TUES WED THUR FRI SAT

	MEALS AND SNACKS	CARB AND FOOD CALCULATIONS	SHOT DETAILS AND LOCATION
BREAKFAST	Total Carbohydrates : ___._ grams	Correction Dose: (BS - ___) / __ (___-___)/__ = (__/__) = ___.__ Carb Dose Calculation: (Meal Carbs / ___) (__._ /___) = ___.__ Correction Dose + Carb Dose Calculation: (_____ + _____) = __.__ OR __ UNITS Correction Dose / Dose Calculation / Rounded to nearest whole number	TIME __ : __ AM / PM LEFT ARM CGM / RIGHT ARM CGM / LEFT LEG CGM / RIGHT LEG CGM / LEFT/RIGHT STOMACH CGM KETONES NEGATIVE / TRACE / SMALL / MODERATE / LARGE
SNACK	Total Carbohydrates : ___._ grams	Carb Dose Calculation: (Meal Carbs / ___) (__._ /___) = ___.__ or __ UNITS NO INSULIN DOSE REQUIRED FOR MEALS/SNACKS UNDER __G OF CARBS OR EQUAL TO __.__ OR LESS	TIME __ : __ AM / PM LEFT ARM CGM / RIGHT ARM CGM / LEFT LEG CGM / RIGHT LEG CGM / LEFT/RIGHT STOMACH CGM KETONES NEGATIVE / TRACE / SMALL / MODERATE / LARGE
LUNCH	Total Carbohydrates : ___._ grams	Correction Dose: (BS - ___) / __ (___-___)/__ = (__/__) = ___.__ Carb Dose Calculation: (Meal Carbs / ___) (__._ /___) = ___.__ Correction Dose + Carb Dose Calculation: (_____ + _____) = __.__ OR __ UNITS Correction Dose / Dose Calculation / Rounded to nearest whole number	TIME __ : __ AM / PM LEFT ARM CGM / RIGHT ARM CGM / LEFT LEG CGM / RIGHT LEG CGM / LEFT/RIGHT STOMACH CGM KETONES NEGATIVE / TRACE / SMALL / MODERATE / LARGE
SNACK	Total Carbohydrates : ___._ grams	Carb Dose Calculation: (Meal Carbs / ___) (__._ /___) = ___.__ or __ UNITS NO INSULIN DOSE REQUIRED FOR MEALS/SNACKS UNDER __G OF CARBS OR EQUAL TO __.__ OR LESS	TIME __ : __ AM / PM LEFT ARM CGM / RIGHT ARM CGM / LEFT LEG CGM / RIGHT LEG CGM / LEFT/RIGHT STOMACH CGM KETONES NEGATIVE / TRACE / SMALL / MODERATE / LARGE
DINNER	Total Carbohydrates : ___._ grams	Correction Dose: (BS - ___) / __ (___-___)/__ = (__/__) = ___.__ Carb Dose Calculation: (Meal Carbs / ___) (__._ /___) = ___.__ Correction Dose + Carb Dose Calculation: (_____ + _____) = __.__ OR __ UNITS Correction Dose / Dose Calculation / Rounded to nearest whole number	TIME __ : __ AM / PM LEFT ARM CGM / RIGHT ARM CGM / LEFT LEG CGM / RIGHT LEG CGM / LEFT/RIGHT STOMACH CGM KETONES NEGATIVE / TRACE / SMALL / MODERATE / LARGE
SNACK	Total Carbohydrates : ___._ grams	Carb Dose Calculation: (Meal Carbs / ___) (__._ /___) = ___.__ or __ UNITS NO INSULIN DOSE REQUIRED FOR MEALS/SNACKS UNDER __G OF CARBS OR EQUAL TO __.__ OR LESS	TIME __ : __ AM / PM LEFT ARM CGM / RIGHT ARM CGM / LEFT LEG CGM / RIGHT LEG CGM / LEFT/RIGHT STOMACH CGM KETONES NEGATIVE / TRACE / SMALL / MODERATE / LARGE
BEDTIME __ : __ PM	BLOOD SUGAR _____ UNITS ___ LEFT ARM CGM / RIGHT ARM CGM / LEFT LEG CGM / RIGHT LEG CGM / LEFT/RIGHT STOMACH CGM KETONES NEGATIVE / TRACE / SMALL / MODERATE / LARGE	HYDRATE 2AM BLOOD SUGAR _____ ADDITIONAL BLOOD SUGAR READINGS BS ___ at __ : __ AM/PM BS ___ at __ : __ AM/PM	NOTES MEDICINE

DATE: ______________________ SUN MON TUES WED THUR FRI SAT

	MEALS AND SNACKS	CARB AND FOOD CALCULATIONS	SHOT DETAILS AND LOCATION
BREAKFAST	Total Carbohydrates : ___._ grams	Correction Dose: (BS - ___) / __ (___-___)/__ = (__/__) = ___.__ Carb Dose Calculation: (Meal Carbs / ___) (__._ /___) = ___.__ Correction Dose + Carb Dose Calculation: (_____ + _____) = __.__ OR __ UNITS Correction Dose · Dose Calculation · Rounded to nearest whole number	TIME __ : __ AM / PM LEFT ARM CGM · RIGHT ARM CGM · LEFT LEG CGM · RIGHT LEG CGM · LEFT/RIGHT STOMACH CGM KETONES NEGATIVE · TRACE · SMALL · MODERATE · LARGE
SNACK	Total Carbohydrates : ___._ grams	Carb Dose Calculation: (Meal Carbs / ___) (__._ /___) = ___.__ or __ UNITS NO INSULIN DOSE REQUIRED FOR MEALS/SNACKS UNDER __G OF CARBS OR EQUAL TO __.__ OR LESS	TIME __ : __ AM / PM LEFT ARM CGM · RIGHT ARM CGM · LEFT LEG CGM · RIGHT LEG CGM · LEFT/RIGHT STOMACH CGM KETONES NEGATIVE · TRACE · SMALL · MODERATE · LARGE
LUNCH	Total Carbohydrates : ___._ grams	Correction Dose: (BS - ___) / __ (___-___)/__ = (__/__) = ___.__ Carb Dose Calculation: (Meal Carbs / ___) (__._ /___) = ___.__ Correction Dose + Carb Dose Calculation: (_____ + _____) = __.__ OR __ UNITS Correction Dose · Dose Calculation · Rounded to nearest whole number	TIME __ : __ AM / PM LEFT ARM CGM · RIGHT ARM CGM · LEFT LEG CGM · RIGHT LEG CGM · LEFT/RIGHT STOMACH CGM KETONES NEGATIVE · TRACE · SMALL · MODERATE · LARGE
SNACK	Total Carbohydrates : ___._ grams	Carb Dose Calculation: (Meal Carbs / ___) (__._ /___) = ___.__ or __ UNITS NO INSULIN DOSE REQUIRED FOR MEALS/SNACKS UNDER __G OF CARBS OR EQUAL TO __.__ OR LESS	TIME __ : __ AM / PM LEFT ARM CGM · RIGHT ARM CGM · LEFT LEG CGM · RIGHT LEG CGM · LEFT/RIGHT STOMACH CGM KETONES NEGATIVE · TRACE · SMALL · MODERATE · LARGE
DINNER	Total Carbohydrates : ___._ grams	Correction Dose: (BS - ___) / __ (___-___)/__ = (__/__) = ___.__ Carb Dose Calculation: (Meal Carbs / ___) (__._ /___) = ___.__ Correction Dose + Carb Dose Calculation: (_____ + _____) = __.__ OR __ UNITS Correction Dose · Dose Calculation · Rounded to nearest whole number	TIME __ : __ AM / PM LEFT ARM CGM · RIGHT ARM CGM · LEFT LEG CGM · RIGHT LEG CGM · LEFT/RIGHT STOMACH CGM KETONES NEGATIVE · TRACE · SMALL · MODERATE · LARGE
SNACK	Total Carbohydrates : ___._ grams	Carb Dose Calculation: (Meal Carbs / ___) (__._ /___) = ___.__ or __ UNITS NO INSULIN DOSE REQUIRED FOR MEALS/SNACKS UNDER __G OF CARBS OR EQUAL TO __.__ OR LESS	TIME __ : __ AM / PM LEFT ARM CGM · RIGHT ARM CGM · LEFT LEG CGM · RIGHT LEG CGM · LEFT/RIGHT STOMACH CGM KETONES NEGATIVE · TRACE · SMALL · MODERATE · LARGE
BEDTIME __ : __ PM	BLOOD SUGAR _____ UNITS ___ LEFT ARM CGM · RIGHT ARM CGM · LEFT LEG CGM · RIGHT LEG CGM · LEFT/RIGHT STOMACH CGM KETONES NEGATIVE · TRACE · SMALL · MODERATE · LARGE	HYDRATE 2AM BLOOD SUGAR _____ ADDITIONAL BLOOD SUGAR READINGS BS ___ at __ : __ AM/PM BS ___ at __ : __ AM/PM	NOTES MEDICINE

DATE: ____________________ SUN MON TUES WED THUR FRI SAT

	MEALS AND SNACKS	CARB AND FOOD CALCULATIONS	SHOT DETAILS AND LOCATION
BREAKFAST	Total Carbohydrates : ___._ grams	Correction Dose: (BS - ___) / __ (___-___)/__ = (__/__) = ___.__ Carb Dose Calculation: (Meal Carbs / ___) (__._ /___) = ___.__ Correction Dose + Carb Dose Calculation: (_____ + _____) = __.__ OR __ UNITS Correction Dose / Dose Calculation / Rounded to nearest whole number	TIME __ : __ AM / PM LEFT ARM CGM / RIGHT ARM CGM / LEFT LEG CGM / RIGHT LEG CGM / LEFT/RIGHT STOMACH CGM KETONES NEGATIVE TRACE SMALL MODERATE LARGE
SNACK	Total Carbohydrates : ___._ grams	Carb Dose Calculation: (Meal Carbs / ___) (__._ /___) = ___.__ or __ UNITS NO INSULIN DOSE REQUIRED FOR MEALS/SNACKS UNDER __G OF CARBS OR EQUAL TO __.__ OR LESS	TIME __ : __ AM / PM LEFT ARM CGM / RIGHT ARM CGM / LEFT LEG CGM / RIGHT LEG CGM / LEFT/RIGHT STOMACH CGM KETONES NEGATIVE TRACE SMALL MODERATE LARGE
LUNCH	Total Carbohydrates : ___._ grams	Correction Dose: (BS - ___) / __ (___-___)/__ = (__/__) = ___.__ Carb Dose Calculation: (Meal Carbs / ___) (__._ /___) = ___.__ Correction Dose + Carb Dose Calculation: (_____ + _____) = __.__ OR __ UNITS Correction Dose / Dose Calculation / Rounded to nearest whole number	TIME __ : __ AM / PM LEFT ARM CGM / RIGHT ARM CGM / LEFT LEG CGM / RIGHT LEG CGM / LEFT/RIGHT STOMACH CGM KETONES NEGATIVE TRACE SMALL MODERATE LARGE
SNACK	Total Carbohydrates : ___._ grams	Carb Dose Calculation: (Meal Carbs / ___) (__._ /___) = ___.__ or __ UNITS NO INSULIN DOSE REQUIRED FOR MEALS/SNACKS UNDER __G OF CARBS OR EQUAL TO __.__ OR LESS	TIME __ : __ AM / PM LEFT ARM CGM / RIGHT ARM CGM / LEFT LEG CGM / RIGHT LEG CGM / LEFT/RIGHT STOMACH CGM KETONES NEGATIVE TRACE SMALL MODERATE LARGE
DINNER	Total Carbohydrates : ___._ grams	Correction Dose: (BS - ___) / __ (___-___)/__ = (__/__) = ___.__ Carb Dose Calculation: (Meal Carbs / ___) (__._ /___) = ___.__ Correction Dose + Carb Dose Calculation: (_____ + _____) = __.__ OR __ UNITS Correction Dose / Dose Calculation / Rounded to nearest whole number	TIME __ : __ AM / PM LEFT ARM CGM / RIGHT ARM CGM / LEFT LEG CGM / RIGHT LEG CGM / LEFT/RIGHT STOMACH CGM KETONES NEGATIVE TRACE SMALL MODERATE LARGE
SNACK	Total Carbohydrates : ___._ grams	Carb Dose Calculation: (Meal Carbs / ___) (__._ /___) = ___.__ or __ UNITS NO INSULIN DOSE REQUIRED FOR MEALS/SNACKS UNDER __G OF CARBS OR EQUAL TO __.__ OR LESS	TIME __ : __ AM / PM LEFT ARM CGM / RIGHT ARM CGM / LEFT LEG CGM / RIGHT LEG CGM / LEFT/RIGHT STOMACH CGM KETONES NEGATIVE TRACE SMALL MODERATE LARGE
BEDTIME __ : __ PM	BLOOD SUGAR _____ UNITS ___ LEFT ARM CGM / RIGHT ARM CGM / LEFT LEG CGM / RIGHT LEG CGM / LEFT/RIGHT STOMACH CGM KETONES NEGATIVE TRACE SMALL MODERATE LARGE	HYDRATE 2AM BLOOD SUGAR _____ ADDITIONAL BLOOD SUGAR READINGS BS ___ at __ : __ AM/PM BS ___ at __ : __ AM/PM	NOTES MEDICINE

DATE: ______________________________ SUN MON TUES WED THUR FRI SAT

	MEALS AND SNACKS	CARB AND FOOD CALCULATIONS	SHOT DETAILS AND LOCATION
BREAKFAST	Total Carbohydrates : ___.__ grams	Correction Dose: (BS - ___) / __ (___-___)/__ = (__/__) = ___.__ Carb Dose Calculation: (Meal Carbs / ___) (__.__ /___) = ___.__ Correction Dose + Carb Dose Calculation: (___.__ + ___.__) = __.__ OR __ UNITS Correction Dose · Dose Calculation · Rounded to nearest whole number	TIME __ : __ AM / PM LEFT ARM CGM · RIGHT ARM CGM · LEFT LEG CGM · RIGHT LEG CGM · LEFT/RIGHT STOMACH CGM KETONES NEGATIVE · TRACE · SMALL · MODERATE · LARGE
SNACK	Total Carbohydrates : ___.__ grams	Carb Dose Calculation: (Meal Carbs / ___) (__.__ /___) = ___.__ or __ UNITS NO INSULIN DOSE REQUIRED FOR MEALS/SNACKS UNDER __G OF CARBS OR EQUAL TO __.__ OR LESS	TIME __ : __ AM / PM LEFT ARM CGM · RIGHT ARM CGM · LEFT LEG CGM · RIGHT LEG CGM · LEFT/RIGHT STOMACH CGM KETONES NEGATIVE · TRACE · SMALL · MODERATE · LARGE
LUNCH	Total Carbohydrates : ___.__ grams	Correction Dose: (BS - ___) / __ (___-___)/__ = (__/__) = ___.__ Carb Dose Calculation: (Meal Carbs / ___) (__.__ /___) = ___.__ Correction Dose + Carb Dose Calculation: (___.__ + ___.__) = __.__ OR __ UNITS Correction Dose · Dose Calculation · Rounded to nearest whole number	TIME __ : __ AM / PM LEFT ARM CGM · RIGHT ARM CGM · LEFT LEG CGM · RIGHT LEG CGM · LEFT/RIGHT STOMACH CGM KETONES NEGATIVE · TRACE · SMALL · MODERATE · LARGE
SNACK	Total Carbohydrates : ___.__ grams	Carb Dose Calculation: (Meal Carbs / ___) (__.__ /___) = ___.__ or __ UNITS NO INSULIN DOSE REQUIRED FOR MEALS/SNACKS UNDER __G OF CARBS OR EQUAL TO __.__ OR LESS	TIME __ : __ AM / PM LEFT ARM CGM · RIGHT ARM CGM · LEFT LEG CGM · RIGHT LEG CGM · LEFT/RIGHT STOMACH CGM KETONES NEGATIVE · TRACE · SMALL · MODERATE · LARGE
DINNER	Total Carbohydrates : ___.__ grams	Correction Dose: (BS - ___) / __ (___-___)/__ = (__/__) = ___.__ Carb Dose Calculation: (Meal Carbs / ___) (__.__ /___) = ___.__ Correction Dose + Carb Dose Calculation: (___.__ + ___.__) = __.__ OR __ UNITS Correction Dose · Dose Calculation · Rounded to nearest whole number	TIME __ : __ AM / PM LEFT ARM CGM · RIGHT ARM CGM · LEFT LEG CGM · RIGHT LEG CGM · LEFT/RIGHT STOMACH CGM KETONES NEGATIVE · TRACE · SMALL · MODERATE · LARGE
SNACK	Total Carbohydrates : ___.__ grams	Carb Dose Calculation: (Meal Carbs / ___) (__.__ /___) = ___.__ or __ UNITS NO INSULIN DOSE REQUIRED FOR MEALS/SNACKS UNDER __G OF CARBS OR EQUAL TO ___.__ OR LESS	TIME __ : __ AM / PM LEFT ARM CGM · RIGHT ARM CGM · LEFT LEG CGM · RIGHT LEG CGM · LEFT/RIGHT STOMACH CGM KETONES NEGATIVE · TRACE · SMALL · MODERATE · LARGE
BEDTIME __ : __ PM	BLOOD SUGAR ____ UNITS ___ LEFT ARM CGM · RIGHT ARM CGM · LEFT LEG CGM · RIGHT LEG CGM · LEFT/RIGHT STOMACH CGM KETONES NEGATIVE · TRACE · SMALL · MODERATE · LARGE	HYDRATE 2AM BLOOD SUGAR ____ ADDITIONAL BLOOD SUGAR READINGS BS ___ at __ : __ AM/PM BS ___ at __ : __ AM/PM	NOTES MEDICINE

DATE: ____________________ SUN MON TUES WED THUR FRI SAT

	MEALS AND SNACKS	CARB AND FOOD CALCULATIONS	SHOT DETAILS AND LOCATION
BREAKFAST	Total Carbohydrates : ___._ grams	Correction Dose: (BS - ___) / __ (___-___)/__ = (__/__) = ___.__ Carb Dose Calculation: (Meal Carbs / ___) (__._ /___) = ___.__ Correction Dose + Carb Dose Calculation: (__.__ + __.__) = __.__ OR __ UNITS Correction Dose / Dose Calculation / Rounded to nearest whole number	TIME __ : __ AM / PM LEFT ARM CGM / RIGHT ARM CGM / LEFT LEG CGM / RIGHT LEG CGM / LEFT/RIGHT STOMACH CGM KETONES NEGATIVE TRACE SMALL MODERATE LARGE
SNACK	Total Carbohydrates : ___._ grams	Carb Dose Calculation: (Meal Carbs / ___) (__._ /___) = ___.__ or __ UNITS NO INSULIN DOSE REQUIRED FOR MEALS/SNACKS UNDER __G OF CARBS OR EQUAL TO __.__ OR LESS	TIME __ : __ AM / PM LEFT ARM CGM / RIGHT ARM CGM / LEFT LEG CGM / RIGHT LEG CGM / LEFT/RIGHT STOMACH CGM KETONES NEGATIVE TRACE SMALL MODERATE LARGE
LUNCH	Total Carbohydrates : ___._ grams	Correction Dose: (BS - ___) / __ (___-___)/__ = (__/__) = ___.__ Carb Dose Calculation: (Meal Carbs / ___) (__._ /___) = ___.__ Correction Dose + Carb Dose Calculation: (__.__ + __.__) = __.__ OR __ UNITS Correction Dose / Dose Calculation / Rounded to nearest whole number	TIME __ : __ AM / PM LEFT ARM CGM / RIGHT ARM CGM / LEFT LEG CGM / RIGHT LEG CGM / LEFT/RIGHT STOMACH CGM KETONES NEGATIVE TRACE SMALL MODERATE LARGE
SNACK	Total Carbohydrates : ___._ grams	Carb Dose Calculation: (Meal Carbs / ___) (__._ /___) = ___.__ or __ UNITS NO INSULIN DOSE REQUIRED FOR MEALS/SNACKS UNDER __G OF CARBS OR EQUAL TO __.__ OR LESS	TIME __ : __ AM / PM LEFT ARM CGM / RIGHT ARM CGM / LEFT LEG CGM / RIGHT LEG CGM / LEFT/RIGHT STOMACH CGM KETONES NEGATIVE TRACE SMALL MODERATE LARGE
DINNER	Total Carbohydrates : ___._ grams	Correction Dose: (BS - ___) / __ (___-___)/__ = (__/__) = ___.__ Carb Dose Calculation: (Meal Carbs / ___) (__._ /___) = ___.__ Correction Dose + Carb Dose Calculation: (__.__ + __.__) = __.__ OR __ UNITS Correction Dose / Dose Calculation / Rounded to nearest whole number	TIME __ : __ AM / PM LEFT ARM CGM / RIGHT ARM CGM / LEFT LEG CGM / RIGHT LEG CGM / LEFT/RIGHT STOMACH CGM KETONES NEGATIVE TRACE SMALL MODERATE LARGE
SNACK	Total Carbohydrates : ___._ grams	Carb Dose Calculation: (Meal Carbs / ___) (__._ /___) = ___.__ or __ UNITS NO INSULIN DOSE REQUIRED FOR MEALS/SNACKS UNDER __G OF CARBS OR EQUAL TO __.__ OR LESS	TIME __ : __ AM / PM LEFT ARM CGM / RIGHT ARM CGM / LEFT LEG CGM / RIGHT LEG CGM / LEFT/RIGHT STOMACH CGM KETONES NEGATIVE TRACE SMALL MODERATE LARGE
BEDTIME __ : __ PM	BLOOD SUGAR ____ UNITS __ LEFT ARM CGM / RIGHT ARM CGM / LEFT LEG CGM / RIGHT LEG CGM / LEFT/RIGHT STOMACH CGM KETONES NEGATIVE TRACE SMALL MODERATE LARGE	HYDRATE 2AM BLOOD SUGAR ____ ADDITIONAL BLOOD SUGAR READINGS BS ___ at __ : __ AM/PM BS ___ at __ : __ AM/PM	NOTES MEDICINE

DATE: ______________________ SUN MON TUES WED THUR FRI SAT

	MEALS AND SNACKS	CARB AND FOOD CALCULATIONS	SHOT DETAILS AND LOCATION
BREAKFAST	Total Carbohydrates : ___.__ grams	Correction Dose: (BS - ___) / __ (___-___)/__ = (__/__) = ___.__ Carb Dose Calculation: (Meal Carbs / ___) (__.__ /___) = ___.__ Correction Dose + Carb Dose Calculation: (_____ + _____) = __.__ OR __ UNITS Correction Dose Dose Calculation Rounded to nearest whole number	TIME __:__ AM / PM LEFT ARM CGM, RIGHT ARM CGM, LEFT LEG CGM, RIGHT LEG CGM, LEFT/RIGHT STOMACH CGM KETONES NEGATIVE TRACE SMALL MODERATE LARGE
SNACK	Total Carbohydrates : ___.__ grams	Carb Dose Calculation: (Meal Carbs / ___) (__.__ /___) = ___.__ or __ UNITS NO INSULIN DOSE REQUIRED FOR MEALS/SNACKS UNDER __G OF CARBS OR EQUAL TO __.__ OR LESS	TIME __:__ AM / PM LEFT ARM CGM, RIGHT ARM CGM, LEFT LEG CGM, RIGHT LEG CGM, LEFT/RIGHT STOMACH CGM KETONES NEGATIVE TRACE SMALL MODERATE LARGE
LUNCH	Total Carbohydrates : ___.__ grams	Correction Dose: (BS - ___) / __ (___-___)/__ = (__/__) = ___.__ Carb Dose Calculation: (Meal Carbs / ___) (__.__ /___) = ___.__ Correction Dose + Carb Dose Calculation: (_____ + _____) = __.__ OR __ UNITS Correction Dose Dose Calculation Rounded to nearest whole number	TIME __:__ AM / PM LEFT ARM CGM, RIGHT ARM CGM, LEFT LEG CGM, RIGHT LEG CGM, LEFT/RIGHT STOMACH CGM KETONES NEGATIVE TRACE SMALL MODERATE LARGE
SNACK	Total Carbohydrates : ___.__ grams	Carb Dose Calculation: (Meal Carbs / ___) (__.__ /___) = ___.__ or __ UNITS NO INSULIN DOSE REQUIRED FOR MEALS/SNACKS UNDER __G OF CARBS OR EQUAL TO __.__ OR LESS	TIME __:__ AM / PM LEFT ARM CGM, RIGHT ARM CGM, LEFT LEG CGM, RIGHT LEG CGM, LEFT/RIGHT STOMACH CGM KETONES NEGATIVE TRACE SMALL MODERATE LARGE
DINNER	Total Carbohydrates : ___.__ grams	Correction Dose: (BS - ___) / __ (___-___)/__ = (__/__) = ___.__ Carb Dose Calculation: (Meal Carbs / ___) (__.__ /___) = ___.__ Correction Dose + Carb Dose Calculation: (_____ + _____) = __.__ OR __ UNITS Correction Dose Dose Calculation Rounded to nearest whole number	TIME __:__ AM / PM LEFT ARM CGM, RIGHT ARM CGM, LEFT LEG CGM, RIGHT LEG CGM, LEFT/RIGHT STOMACH CGM KETONES NEGATIVE TRACE SMALL MODERATE LARGE
SNACK	Total Carbohydrates : ___.__ grams	Carb Dose Calculation: (Meal Carbs / ___) (__.__ /___) = ___.__ or __ UNITS NO INSULIN DOSE REQUIRED FOR MEALS/SNACKS UNDER __G OF CARBS OR EQUAL TO __.__ OR LESS	TIME __:__ AM / PM LEFT ARM CGM, RIGHT ARM CGM, LEFT LEG CGM, RIGHT LEG CGM, LEFT/RIGHT STOMACH CGM KETONES NEGATIVE TRACE SMALL MODERATE LARGE
BEDTIME __:__ PM	BLOOD SUGAR _____ UNITS ___ LEFT ARM CGM, RIGHT ARM CGM, LEFT LEG CGM, RIGHT LEG CGM, LEFT/RIGHT STOMACH CGM KETONES NEGATIVE TRACE SMALL MODERATE LARGE	HYDRATE 2AM BLOOD SUGAR _____ ADDITIONAL BLOOD SUGAR READINGS BS ___ at __ : __ AM/PM BS ___ at __ : __ AM/PM	NOTES MEDICINE

DATE: ____________________ SUN MON TUES WED THUR FRI SAT

	MEALS AND SNACKS	CARB AND FOOD CALCULATIONS	SHOT DETAILS AND LOCATION
BREAKFAST	Total Carbohydrates : ___._ grams	Correction Dose: (BS - ___) / __ (___-___)/__ = (__/__) = ___.__ Carb Dose Calculation: (Meal Carbs / ___) (__._ /___) = ___.__ Correction Dose + Carb Dose Calculation: (__.__ + __.__) = __.__ OR __ UNITS Correction Dose / Dose Calculation / Rounded to nearest whole number	TIME __ : __ AM / PM LEFT ARM CGM / RIGHT ARM CGM / LEFT LEG CGM / RIGHT LEG CGM / LEFT/RIGHT STOMACH CGM KETONES NEGATIVE / TRACE / SMALL / MODERATE / LARGE
SNACK	Total Carbohydrates : ___._ grams	Carb Dose Calculation: (Meal Carbs / ___) (__._ /___) = ___.__ or __ UNITS NO INSULIN DOSE REQUIRED FOR MEALS/SNACKS UNDER __G OF CARBS OR EQUAL TO __.__ OR LESS	TIME __ : __ AM / PM LEFT ARM CGM / RIGHT ARM CGM / LEFT LEG CGM / RIGHT LEG CGM / LEFT/RIGHT STOMACH CGM KETONES NEGATIVE / TRACE / SMALL / MODERATE / LARGE
LUNCH	Total Carbohydrates : ___._ grams	Correction Dose: (BS - ___) / __ (___-___)/__ = (__/__) = ___.__ Carb Dose Calculation: (Meal Carbs / ___) (__._ /___) = ___.__ Correction Dose + Carb Dose Calculation: (__.__ + __.__) = __.__ OR __ UNITS Correction Dose / Dose Calculation / Rounded to nearest whole number	TIME __ : __ AM / PM LEFT ARM CGM / RIGHT ARM CGM / LEFT LEG CGM / RIGHT LEG CGM / LEFT/RIGHT STOMACH CGM KETONES NEGATIVE / TRACE / SMALL / MODERATE / LARGE
SNACK	Total Carbohydrates : ___._ grams	Carb Dose Calculation: (Meal Carbs / ___) (__._ /___) = ___.__ or __ UNITS NO INSULIN DOSE REQUIRED FOR MEALS/SNACKS UNDER __G OF CARBS OR EQUAL TO __.__ OR LESS	TIME __ : __ AM / PM LEFT ARM CGM / RIGHT ARM CGM / LEFT LEG CGM / RIGHT LEG CGM / LEFT/RIGHT STOMACH CGM KETONES NEGATIVE / TRACE / SMALL / MODERATE / LARGE
DINNER	Total Carbohydrates : ___._ grams	Correction Dose: (BS - ___) / __ (___-___)/__ = (__/__) = ___.__ Carb Dose Calculation: (Meal Carbs / ___) (__._ /___) = ___.__ Correction Dose + Carb Dose Calculation: (__.__ + __.__) = __.__ OR __ UNITS Correction Dose / Dose Calculation / Rounded to nearest whole number	TIME __ : __ AM / PM LEFT ARM CGM / RIGHT ARM CGM / LEFT LEG CGM / RIGHT LEG CGM / LEFT/RIGHT STOMACH CGM KETONES NEGATIVE / TRACE / SMALL / MODERATE / LARGE
SNACK	Total Carbohydrates : ___._ grams	Carb Dose Calculation: (Meal Carbs / ___) (__._ /___) = ___.__ or __ UNITS NO INSULIN DOSE REQUIRED FOR MEALS/SNACKS UNDER __G OF CARBS OR EQUAL TO __.__ OR LESS	TIME __ : __ AM / PM LEFT ARM CGM / RIGHT ARM CGM / LEFT LEG CGM / RIGHT LEG CGM / LEFT/RIGHT STOMACH CGM KETONES NEGATIVE / TRACE / SMALL / MODERATE / LARGE
BEDTIME __ : __ PM	BLOOD SUGAR ____ UNITS ___ LEFT ARM CGM / RIGHT ARM CGM / LEFT LEG CGM / RIGHT LEG CGM / LEFT/RIGHT STOMACH CGM KETONES NEGATIVE / TRACE / SMALL / MODERATE / LARGE	HYDRATE 2AM BLOOD SUGAR ____ ADDITIONAL BLOOD SUGAR READINGS BS ___ at __ : __ AM/PM BS ___ at __ : __ AM/PM	NOTES MEDICINE

DATE: ______________________________ SUN MON TUES WED THUR FRI SAT

	MEALS AND SNACKS	CARB AND FOOD CALCULATIONS	SHOT DETAILS AND LOCATION
BREAKFAST	Total Carbohydrates : ___._ grams	Correction Dose: (BS - ___) / __ (___-___)/__ = (__/__) = ___.__ Carb Dose Calculation: (Meal Carbs / ___) (__._ /___) = ___.__ Correction Dose + Carb Dose Calculation: (__.__ + __.__) = __.__ OR __ UNITS Correction Dose / Dose Calculation / Rounded to nearest whole number	TIME __ : __ AM / PM LEFT ARM CGM / RIGHT ARM CGM / LEFT LEG CGM / RIGHT LEG CGM / LEFT/RIGHT STOMACH CGM KETONES NEGATIVE / TRACE / SMALL / MODERATE / LARGE
SNACK	Total Carbohydrates : ___._ grams	Carb Dose Calculation: (Meal Carbs / ___) (__._ /___) = ___.__ or __ UNITS NO INSULIN DOSE REQUIRED FOR MEALS/SNACKS UNDER __G OF CARBS OR EQUAL TO __.__ OR LESS	TIME __ : __ AM / PM LEFT ARM CGM / RIGHT ARM CGM / LEFT LEG CGM / RIGHT LEG CGM / LEFT/RIGHT STOMACH CGM KETONES NEGATIVE / TRACE / SMALL / MODERATE / LARGE
LUNCH	Total Carbohydrates : ___._ grams	Correction Dose: (BS - ___) / __ (___-___)/__ = (__/__) = ___.__ Carb Dose Calculation: (Meal Carbs / ___) (__._ /___) = ___.__ Correction Dose + Carb Dose Calculation: (__.__ + __.__) = __.__ OR __ UNITS Correction Dose / Dose Calculation / Rounded to nearest whole number	TIME __ : __ AM / PM LEFT ARM CGM / RIGHT ARM CGM / LEFT LEG CGM / RIGHT LEG CGM / LEFT/RIGHT STOMACH CGM KETONES NEGATIVE / TRACE / SMALL / MODERATE / LARGE
SNACK	Total Carbohydrates : ___._ grams	Carb Dose Calculation: (Meal Carbs / ___) (__._ /___) = ___.__ or __ UNITS NO INSULIN DOSE REQUIRED FOR MEALS/SNACKS UNDER __G OF CARBS OR EQUAL TO __.__ OR LESS	TIME __ : __ AM / PM LEFT ARM CGM / RIGHT ARM CGM / LEFT LEG CGM / RIGHT LEG CGM / LEFT/RIGHT STOMACH CGM KETONES NEGATIVE / TRACE / SMALL / MODERATE / LARGE
DINNER	Total Carbohydrates : ___._ grams	Correction Dose: (BS - ___) / __ (___-___)/__ = (__/__) = ___.__ Carb Dose Calculation: (Meal Carbs / ___) (__._ /___) = ___.__ Correction Dose + Carb Dose Calculation: (__.__ + __.__) = __.__ OR __ UNITS Correction Dose / Dose Calculation / Rounded to nearest whole number	TIME __ : __ AM / PM LEFT ARM CGM / RIGHT ARM CGM / LEFT LEG CGM / RIGHT LEG CGM / LEFT/RIGHT STOMACH CGM KETONES NEGATIVE / TRACE / SMALL / MODERATE / LARGE
SNACK	Total Carbohydrates : ___._ grams	Carb Dose Calculation: (Meal Carbs / ___) (__._ /___) = ___.__ or __ UNITS NO INSULIN DOSE REQUIRED FOR MEALS/SNACKS UNDER __G OF CARBS OR EQUAL TO __.__ OR LESS	TIME __ : __ AM / PM LEFT ARM CGM / RIGHT ARM CGM / LEFT LEG CGM / RIGHT LEG CGM / LEFT/RIGHT STOMACH CGM KETONES NEGATIVE / TRACE / SMALL / MODERATE / LARGE
BEDTIME __ : __ PM	BLOOD SUGAR ____ UNITS ___ LEFT ARM CGM / RIGHT ARM CGM / LEFT LEG CGM / RIGHT LEG CGM / LEFT/RIGHT STOMACH CGM KETONES NEGATIVE / TRACE / SMALL / MODERATE / LARGE	HYDRATE 2AM BLOOD SUGAR ____ ADDITIONAL BLOOD SUGAR READINGS BS ___ at __ : __ AM/PM BS ___ at __ : __ AM/PM	NOTES MEDICINE

DATE: ______________________________ SUN MON TUES WED THUR FRI SAT

	MEALS AND SNACKS	CARB AND FOOD CALCULATIONS	SHOT DETAILS AND LOCATION
BREAKFAST	Total Carbohydrates : ___._ grams	Correction Dose: (BS - ___) / __ (___-___)/__ = (__/__) = ___.__ Carb Dose Calculation: (Meal Carbs / ___) (__._ /___) = ___.__ Correction Dose + Carb Dose Calculation: (_____ + _____) = __.__ OR __ UNITS Correction Dose / Dose Calculation / Rounded to nearest whole number	TIME __ : __ AM / PM LEFT ARM CGM / RIGHT ARM CGM / LEFT LEG CGM / RIGHT LEG CGM / LEFT/RIGHT STOMACH CGM KETONES NEGATIVE / TRACE / SMALL / MODERATE / LARGE
SNACK	Total Carbohydrates : ___._ grams	Carb Dose Calculation: (Meal Carbs / ___) (__._ /___) = ___.__ or __ UNITS NO INSULIN DOSE REQUIRED FOR MEALS/SNACKS UNDER __G OF CARBS OR EQUAL TO __.__ OR LESS	TIME __ : __ AM / PM LEFT ARM CGM / RIGHT ARM CGM / LEFT LEG CGM / RIGHT LEG CGM / LEFT/RIGHT STOMACH CGM KETONES NEGATIVE / TRACE / SMALL / MODERATE / LARGE
LUNCH	Total Carbohydrates : ___._ grams	Correction Dose: (BS - ___) / __ (___-___)/__ = (__/__) = ___.__ Carb Dose Calculation: (Meal Carbs / ___) (__._ /___) = ___.__ Correction Dose + Carb Dose Calculation: (_____ + _____) = __.__ OR __ UNITS Correction Dose / Dose Calculation / Rounded to nearest whole number	TIME __ : __ AM / PM LEFT ARM CGM / RIGHT ARM CGM / LEFT LEG CGM / RIGHT LEG CGM / LEFT/RIGHT STOMACH CGM KETONES NEGATIVE / TRACE / SMALL / MODERATE / LARGE
SNACK	Total Carbohydrates : ___._ grams	Carb Dose Calculation: (Meal Carbs / ___) (__._ /___) = ___.__ or __ UNITS NO INSULIN DOSE REQUIRED FOR MEALS/SNACKS UNDER __G OF CARBS OR EQUAL TO __.__ OR LESS	TIME __ : __ AM / PM LEFT ARM CGM / RIGHT ARM CGM / LEFT LEG CGM / RIGHT LEG CGM / LEFT/RIGHT STOMACH CGM KETONES NEGATIVE / TRACE / SMALL / MODERATE / LARGE
DINNER	Total Carbohydrates : ___._ grams	Correction Dose: (BS - ___) / __ (___-___)/__ = (__/__) = ___.__ Carb Dose Calculation: (Meal Carbs / ___) (__._ /___) = ___.__ Correction Dose + Carb Dose Calculation: (_____ + _____) = __.__ OR __ UNITS Correction Dose / Dose Calculation / Rounded to nearest whole number	TIME __ : __ AM / PM LEFT ARM CGM / RIGHT ARM CGM / LEFT LEG CGM / RIGHT LEG CGM / LEFT/RIGHT STOMACH CGM KETONES NEGATIVE / TRACE / SMALL / MODERATE / LARGE
SNACK	Total Carbohydrates : ___._ grams	Carb Dose Calculation: (Meal Carbs / ___) (__._ /___) = ___.__ or __ UNITS NO INSULIN DOSE REQUIRED FOR MEALS/SNACKS UNDER __G OF CARBS OR EQUAL TO __.__ OR LESS	TIME __ : __ AM / PM LEFT ARM CGM / RIGHT ARM CGM / LEFT LEG CGM / RIGHT LEG CGM / LEFT/RIGHT STOMACH CGM KETONES NEGATIVE / TRACE / SMALL / MODERATE / LARGE
BEDTIME __ : __ PM	BLOOD SUGAR _____ UNITS ___ LEFT ARM CGM / RIGHT ARM CGM / LEFT LEG CGM / RIGHT LEG CGM / LEFT/RIGHT STOMACH CGM KETONES NEGATIVE / TRACE / SMALL / MODERATE / LARGE	HYDRATE 2AM BLOOD SUGAR _____ ADDITIONAL BLOOD SUGAR READINGS BS ___ at __ : __ AM/PM BS ___ at __ : __ AM/PM	NOTES MEDICINE

DATE: ____________________ SUN MON TUES WED THUR FRI SAT

	MEALS AND SNACKS	CARB AND FOOD CALCULATIONS	SHOT DETAILS AND LOCATION
BREAKFAST	Total Carbohydrates : ___._ grams	Correction Dose: (BS - ___) / __ (___-___)/__ = (__/__) = ___.__ Carb Dose Calculation: (Meal Carbs / ___) (__._ /___) = ___.__ Correction Dose + Carb Dose Calculation: (___.__ + ___.__) = __.__ OR __ UNITS Correction Dose / Dose Calculation / Rounded to nearest whole number	TIME __ :__ AM / PM LEFT ARM CGM / RIGHT ARM CGM / LEFT LEG CGM / RIGHT LEG CGM / LEFT/RIGHT STOMACH CGM KETONES NEGATIVE / TRACE / SMALL / MODERATE / LARGE
SNACK	Total Carbohydrates : ___._ grams	Carb Dose Calculation: (Meal Carbs / ___) (__._ /___) = ___.__ or __ UNITS NO INSULIN DOSE REQUIRED FOR MEALS/SNACKS UNDER __G OF CARBS OR EQUAL TO __.__ OR LESS	TIME __ :__ AM / PM LEFT ARM CGM / RIGHT ARM CGM / LEFT LEG CGM / RIGHT LEG CGM / LEFT/RIGHT STOMACH CGM KETONES NEGATIVE / TRACE / SMALL / MODERATE / LARGE
LUNCH	Total Carbohydrates : ___._ grams	Correction Dose: (BS - ___) / __ (___-___)/__ = (__/__) = ___.__ Carb Dose Calculation: (Meal Carbs / ___) (__._ /___) = ___.__ Correction Dose + Carb Dose Calculation: (___.__ + ___.__) = __.__ OR __ UNITS Correction Dose / Dose Calculation / Rounded to nearest whole number	TIME __ :__ AM / PM LEFT ARM CGM / RIGHT ARM CGM / LEFT LEG CGM / RIGHT LEG CGM / LEFT/RIGHT STOMACH CGM KETONES NEGATIVE / TRACE / SMALL / MODERATE / LARGE
SNACK	Total Carbohydrates : ___._ grams	Carb Dose Calculation: (Meal Carbs / ___) (__._ /___) = ___.__ or __ UNITS NO INSULIN DOSE REQUIRED FOR MEALS/SNACKS UNDER __G OF CARBS OR EQUAL TO __.__ OR LESS	TIME __ :__ AM / PM LEFT ARM CGM / RIGHT ARM CGM / LEFT LEG CGM / RIGHT LEG CGM / LEFT/RIGHT STOMACH CGM KETONES NEGATIVE / TRACE / SMALL / MODERATE / LARGE
DINNER	Total Carbohydrates : ___._ grams	Correction Dose: (BS - ___) / __ (___-___)/__ = (__/__) = ___.__ Carb Dose Calculation: (Meal Carbs / ___) (__._ /___) = ___.__ Correction Dose + Carb Dose Calculation: (___.__ + ___.__) = __.__ OR __ UNITS Correction Dose / Dose Calculation / Rounded to nearest whole number	TIME __ :__ AM / PM LEFT ARM CGM / RIGHT ARM CGM / LEFT LEG CGM / RIGHT LEG CGM / LEFT/RIGHT STOMACH CGM KETONES NEGATIVE / TRACE / SMALL / MODERATE / LARGE
SNACK	Total Carbohydrates : ___._ grams	Carb Dose Calculation: (Meal Carbs / ___) (__._ /___) = ___.__ or __ UNITS NO INSULIN DOSE REQUIRED FOR MEALS/SNACKS UNDER __G OF CARBS OR EQUAL TO __.__ OR LESS	TIME __ :__ AM / PM LEFT ARM CGM / RIGHT ARM CGM / LEFT LEG CGM / RIGHT LEG CGM / LEFT/RIGHT STOMACH CGM KETONES NEGATIVE / TRACE / SMALL / MODERATE / LARGE
BEDTIME __ : __ PM	BLOOD SUGAR _____ UNITS ___ LEFT ARM CGM / RIGHT ARM CGM / LEFT LEG CGM / RIGHT LEG CGM / LEFT/RIGHT STOMACH CGM KETONES NEGATIVE / TRACE / SMALL / MODERATE / LARGE	HYDRATE 2AM BLOOD SUGAR _____ ADDITIONAL BLOOD SUGAR READINGS BS ___ at __ : __ AM/PM BS ___ at __ : __ AM/PM	NOTES MEDICINE

DATE: ______________________ SUN MON TUES WED THUR FRI SAT

	MEALS AND SNACKS	CARB AND FOOD CALCULATIONS	SHOT DETAILS AND LOCATION
BREAKFAST	Total Carbohydrates : ___._ grams	Correction Dose: (BS - ___) / __ (___-___)/__ = (__/__) = ___.__ Carb Dose Calculation: (Meal Carbs / ___) (__._ /___) = ___.__ Correction Dose + Carb Dose Calculation: (___.__ + ___.__) = ___.__ OR __ UNITS Correction Dose / Dose Calculation / Rounded to nearest whole number	TIME __ : __ AM / PM LEFT ARM CGM / RIGHT ARM CGM / LEFT LEG CGM / RIGHT LEG CGM / LEFT/RIGHT STOMACH CGM KETONES NEGATIVE / TRACE / SMALL / MODERATE / LARGE
SNACK	Total Carbohydrates : ___._ grams	Carb Dose Calculation: (Meal Carbs / ___) (__._ /___) = ___.__ or __ UNITS NO INSULIN DOSE REQUIRED FOR MEALS/SNACKS UNDER __G OF CARBS OR EQUAL TO __.__ OR LESS	TIME __ : __ AM / PM LEFT ARM CGM / RIGHT ARM CGM / LEFT LEG CGM / RIGHT LEG CGM / LEFT/RIGHT STOMACH CGM KETONES NEGATIVE / TRACE / SMALL / MODERATE / LARGE
LUNCH	Total Carbohydrates : ___._ grams	Correction Dose: (BS - ___) / __ (___-___)/__ = (__/__) = ___.__ Carb Dose Calculation: (Meal Carbs / ___) (__._ /___) = ___.__ Correction Dose + Carb Dose Calculation: (___.__ + ___.__) = ___.__ OR __ UNITS Correction Dose / Dose Calculation / Rounded to nearest whole number	TIME __ : __ AM / PM LEFT ARM CGM / RIGHT ARM CGM / LEFT LEG CGM / RIGHT LEG CGM / LEFT/RIGHT STOMACH CGM KETONES NEGATIVE / TRACE / SMALL / MODERATE / LARGE
SNACK	Total Carbohydrates : ___._ grams	Carb Dose Calculation: (Meal Carbs / ___) (__._ /___) = ___.__ or __ UNITS NO INSULIN DOSE REQUIRED FOR MEALS/SNACKS UNDER __G OF CARBS OR EQUAL TO __.__ OR LESS	TIME __ : __ AM / PM LEFT ARM CGM / RIGHT ARM CGM / LEFT LEG CGM / RIGHT LEG CGM / LEFT/RIGHT STOMACH CGM KETONES NEGATIVE / TRACE / SMALL / MODERATE / LARGE
DINNER	Total Carbohydrates : ___._ grams	Correction Dose: (BS - ___) / __ (___-___)/__ = (__/__) = ___.__ Carb Dose Calculation: (Meal Carbs / ___) (__._ /___) = ___.__ Correction Dose + Carb Dose Calculation: (___.__ + ___.__) = ___.__ OR __ UNITS Correction Dose / Dose Calculation / Rounded to nearest whole number	TIME __ : __ AM / PM LEFT ARM CGM / RIGHT ARM CGM / LEFT LEG CGM / RIGHT LEG CGM / LEFT/RIGHT STOMACH CGM KETONES NEGATIVE / TRACE / SMALL / MODERATE / LARGE
SNACK	Total Carbohydrates : ___._ grams	Carb Dose Calculation: (Meal Carbs / ___) (__._ /___) = ___.__ or __ UNITS NO INSULIN DOSE REQUIRED FOR MEALS/SNACKS UNDER __G OF CARBS OR EQUAL TO __.__ OR LESS	TIME __ : __ AM / PM LEFT ARM CGM / RIGHT ARM CGM / LEFT LEG CGM / RIGHT LEG CGM / LEFT/RIGHT STOMACH CGM KETONES NEGATIVE / TRACE / SMALL / MODERATE / LARGE
BEDTIME __ : __ PM	BLOOD SUGAR ____ UNITS ___ LEFT ARM CGM / RIGHT ARM CGM / LEFT LEG CGM / RIGHT LEG CGM / LEFT/RIGHT STOMACH CGM KETONES NEGATIVE / TRACE / SMALL / MODERATE / LARGE	HYDRATE 2AM BLOOD SUGAR ____ ADDITIONAL BLOOD SUGAR READINGS BS ___ at __ : __ AM/PM BS ___ at __ : __ AM/PM	NOTES MEDICINE

DATE: ____________________ SUN MON TUES WED THUR FRI SAT

	MEALS AND SNACKS	CARB AND FOOD CALCULATIONS	SHOT DETAILS AND LOCATION
BREAKFAST	Total Carbohydrates : ___._ grams	Correction Dose: (BS - ___) / __ (___-___)/__ = (__/__) = ___.__ Carb Dose Calculation: (Meal Carbs / ___) (__._ /___) = ___.__ Correction Dose + Carb Dose Calculation: (______ + ______) = __.__ OR __ UNITS Correction Dose / Dose Calculation / Rounded to nearest whole number	TIME __ : __ AM / PM LEFT ARM CGM / RIGHT ARM CGM / LEFT LEG CGM / RIGHT LEG CGM / LEFT/RIGHT STOMACH CGM KETONES NEGATIVE / TRACE / SMALL / MODERATE / LARGE
SNACK	Total Carbohydrates : ___._ grams	Carb Dose Calculation: (Meal Carbs / ___) (__._ /___) = ___.__ or __ UNITS NO INSULIN DOSE REQUIRED FOR MEALS/SNACKS UNDER __G OF CARBS OR EQUAL TO __.__ OR LESS	TIME __ : __ AM / PM LEFT ARM CGM / RIGHT ARM CGM / LEFT LEG CGM / RIGHT LEG CGM / LEFT/RIGHT STOMACH CGM KETONES NEGATIVE / TRACE / SMALL / MODERATE / LARGE
LUNCH	Total Carbohydrates : ___._ grams	Correction Dose: (BS - ___) / __ (___-___)/__ = (__/__) = ___.__ Carb Dose Calculation: (Meal Carbs / ___) (__._ /___) = ___.__ Correction Dose + Carb Dose Calculation: (______ + ______) = __.__ OR __ UNITS Correction Dose / Dose Calculation / Rounded to nearest whole number	TIME __ : __ AM / PM LEFT ARM CGM / RIGHT ARM CGM / LEFT LEG CGM / RIGHT LEG CGM / LEFT/RIGHT STOMACH CGM KETONES NEGATIVE / TRACE / SMALL / MODERATE / LARGE
SNACK	Total Carbohydrates : ___._ grams	Carb Dose Calculation: (Meal Carbs / ___) (__._ /___) = ___.__ or __ UNITS NO INSULIN DOSE REQUIRED FOR MEALS/SNACKS UNDER __G OF CARBS OR EQUAL TO __.__ OR LESS	TIME __ : __ AM / PM LEFT ARM CGM / RIGHT ARM CGM / LEFT LEG CGM / RIGHT LEG CGM / LEFT/RIGHT STOMACH CGM KETONES NEGATIVE / TRACE / SMALL / MODERATE / LARGE
DINNER	Total Carbohydrates : ___._ grams	Correction Dose: (BS - ___) / __ (___-___)/__ = (__/__) = ___.__ Carb Dose Calculation: (Meal Carbs / ___) (__._ /___) = ___.__ Correction Dose + Carb Dose Calculation: (______ + ______) = __.__ OR __ UNITS Correction Dose / Dose Calculation / Rounded to nearest whole number	TIME __ : __ AM / PM LEFT ARM CGM / RIGHT ARM CGM / LEFT LEG CGM / RIGHT LEG CGM / LEFT/RIGHT STOMACH CGM KETONES NEGATIVE / TRACE / SMALL / MODERATE / LARGE
SNACK	Total Carbohydrates : ___._ grams	Carb Dose Calculation: (Meal Carbs / ___) (__._ /___) = ___.__ or __ UNITS NO INSULIN DOSE REQUIRED FOR MEALS/SNACKS UNDER __G OF CARBS OR EQUAL TO __.__ OR LESS	TIME __ : __ AM / PM LEFT ARM CGM / RIGHT ARM CGM / LEFT LEG CGM / RIGHT LEG CGM / LEFT/RIGHT STOMACH CGM KETONES NEGATIVE / TRACE / SMALL / MODERATE / LARGE
BEDTIME __ : __ PM	BLOOD SUGAR _____ UNITS ___ LEFT ARM CGM / RIGHT ARM CGM / LEFT LEG CGM / RIGHT LEG CGM / LEFT/RIGHT STOMACH CGM KETONES NEGATIVE / TRACE / SMALL / MODERATE / LARGE	HYDRATE 2AM BLOOD SUGAR _____ ADDITIONAL BLOOD SUGAR READINGS BS ___ at __ : __ AM/PM BS ___ at __ : __ AM/PM	NOTES MEDICINE

DATE: ______________________ SUN MON TUES WED THUR FRI SAT

	MEALS AND SNACKS	CARB AND FOOD CALCULATIONS	SHOT DETAILS AND LOCATION
BREAKFAST	Total Carbohydrates : ___._ grams	Correction Dose: (BS - ___) / __ (___-___)/__ = (__/__) = ___.__ Carb Dose Calculation: (Meal Carbs / ___) (__._ /___) = ___.__ Correction Dose + Carb Dose Calculation: (_____ + _____) = __.__ OR __ UNITS Correction Dose Dose Calculation Rounded to nearest whole number	TIME __ : __ AM / PM LEFT ARM CGM / RIGHT ARM CGM / LEFT LEG CGM / RIGHT LEG CGM / LEFT/RIGHT STOMACH CGM KETONES NEGATIVE TRACE SMALL MODERATE LARGE
SNACK	Total Carbohydrates : ___._ grams	Carb Dose Calculation: (Meal Carbs / ___) (__._ /___) = ___.__ or __ UNITS NO INSULIN DOSE REQUIRED FOR MEALS/SNACKS UNDER __G OF CARBS OR EQUAL TO __.__ OR LESS	TIME __ : __ AM / PM LEFT ARM CGM / RIGHT ARM CGM / LEFT LEG CGM / RIGHT LEG CGM / LEFT/RIGHT STOMACH CGM KETONES NEGATIVE TRACE SMALL MODERATE LARGE
LUNCH	Total Carbohydrates : ___._ grams	Correction Dose: (BS - ___) / __ (___-___)/__ = (__/__) = ___.__ Carb Dose Calculation: (Meal Carbs / ___) (__._ /___) = ___.__ Correction Dose + Carb Dose Calculation: (_____ + _____) = __.__ OR __ UNITS Correction Dose Dose Calculation Rounded to nearest whole number	TIME __ : __ AM / PM LEFT ARM CGM / RIGHT ARM CGM / LEFT LEG CGM / RIGHT LEG CGM / LEFT/RIGHT STOMACH CGM KETONES NEGATIVE TRACE SMALL MODERATE LARGE
SNACK	Total Carbohydrates : ___._ grams	Carb Dose Calculation: (Meal Carbs / ___) (__._ /___) = ___.__ or __ UNITS NO INSULIN DOSE REQUIRED FOR MEALS/SNACKS UNDER __G OF CARBS OR EQUAL TO __.__ OR LESS	TIME __ : __ AM / PM LEFT ARM CGM / RIGHT ARM CGM / LEFT LEG CGM / RIGHT LEG CGM / LEFT/RIGHT STOMACH CGM KETONES NEGATIVE TRACE SMALL MODERATE LARGE
DINNER	Total Carbohydrates : ___._ grams	Correction Dose: (BS - ___) / __ (___-___)/__ = (__/__) = ___.__ Carb Dose Calculation: (Meal Carbs / ___) (__._ /___) = ___.__ Correction Dose + Carb Dose Calculation: (_____ + _____) = __.__ OR __ UNITS Correction Dose Dose Calculation Rounded to nearest whole number	TIME __ : __ AM / PM LEFT ARM CGM / RIGHT ARM CGM / LEFT LEG CGM / RIGHT LEG CGM / LEFT/RIGHT STOMACH CGM KETONES NEGATIVE TRACE SMALL MODERATE LARGE
SNACK	Total Carbohydrates : ___._ grams	Carb Dose Calculation: (Meal Carbs / ___) (__._ /___) = ___.__ or __ UNITS NO INSULIN DOSE REQUIRED FOR MEALS/SNACKS UNDER __G OF CARBS OR EQUAL TO __.__ OR LESS	TIME __ : __ AM / PM LEFT ARM CGM / RIGHT ARM CGM / LEFT LEG CGM / RIGHT LEG CGM / LEFT/RIGHT STOMACH CGM KETONES NEGATIVE TRACE SMALL MODERATE LARGE
BEDTIME __ : __ PM	BLOOD SUGAR ____ UNITS ___ LEFT ARM CGM / RIGHT ARM CGM / LEFT LEG CGM / RIGHT LEG CGM / LEFT/RIGHT STOMACH CGM KETONES NEGATIVE TRACE SMALL MODERATE LARGE	HYDRATE 2AM BLOOD SUGAR ____ ADDITIONAL BLOOD SUGAR READINGS BS ___ at __ : __ AM/PM BS ___ at __ : __ AM/PM	NOTES MEDICINE

DATE: ______________________ SUN MON TUES WED THUR FRI SAT

	MEALS AND SNACKS	CARB AND FOOD CALCULATIONS	SHOT DETAILS AND LOCATION
BREAKFAST	Total Carbohydrates : ___._ grams	Correction Dose: (BS - ___) / __ (___-___)/__ = (__/__) = ___.__ Carb Dose Calculation: (Meal Carbs / ___) (__._ /___) = ___.__ Correction Dose + Carb Dose Calculation: (_____ + _____) = __.__ OR __ UNITS Correction Dose / Dose Calculation / Rounded to nearest whole number	TIME __ :__ AM / PM LEFT ARM CGM / RIGHT ARM CGM / LEFT LEG CGM / RIGHT LEG CGM / LEFT/RIGHT STOMACH CGM KETONES NEGATIVE / TRACE / SMALL / MODERATE / LARGE
SNACK	Total Carbohydrates : ___._ grams	Carb Dose Calculation: (Meal Carbs / ___) (__._ /___) = ___.__ or __ UNITS NO INSULIN DOSE REQUIRED FOR MEALS/SNACKS UNDER __G OF CARBS OR EQUAL TO __.__ OR LESS	TIME __ :__ AM / PM LEFT ARM CGM / RIGHT ARM CGM / LEFT LEG CGM / RIGHT LEG CGM / LEFT/RIGHT STOMACH CGM KETONES NEGATIVE / TRACE / SMALL / MODERATE / LARGE
LUNCH	Total Carbohydrates : ___._ grams	Correction Dose: (BS - ___) / __ (___-___)/__ = (__/__) = ___.__ Carb Dose Calculation: (Meal Carbs / ___) (__._ /___) = ___.__ Correction Dose + Carb Dose Calculation: (_____ + _____) = __.__ OR __ UNITS Correction Dose / Dose Calculation / Rounded to nearest whole number	TIME __ :__ AM / PM LEFT ARM CGM / RIGHT ARM CGM / LEFT LEG CGM / RIGHT LEG CGM / LEFT/RIGHT STOMACH CGM KETONES NEGATIVE / TRACE / SMALL / MODERATE / LARGE
SNACK	Total Carbohydrates : ___._ grams	Carb Dose Calculation: (Meal Carbs / ___) (__._ /___) = ___.__ or __ UNITS NO INSULIN DOSE REQUIRED FOR MEALS/SNACKS UNDER __G OF CARBS OR EQUAL TO __.__ OR LESS	TIME __ :__ AM / PM LEFT ARM CGM / RIGHT ARM CGM / LEFT LEG CGM / RIGHT LEG CGM / LEFT/RIGHT STOMACH CGM KETONES NEGATIVE / TRACE / SMALL / MODERATE / LARGE
DINNER	Total Carbohydrates : ___._ grams	Correction Dose: (BS - ___) / __ (___-___)/__ = (__/__) = ___.__ Carb Dose Calculation: (Meal Carbs / ___) (__._ /___) = ___.__ Correction Dose + Carb Dose Calculation: (_____ + _____) = __.__ OR __ UNITS Correction Dose / Dose Calculation / Rounded to nearest whole number	TIME __ :__ AM / PM LEFT ARM CGM / RIGHT ARM CGM / LEFT LEG CGM / RIGHT LEG CGM / LEFT/RIGHT STOMACH CGM KETONES NEGATIVE / TRACE / SMALL / MODERATE / LARGE
SNACK	Total Carbohydrates : ___._ grams	Carb Dose Calculation: (Meal Carbs / ___) (__._ /___) = ___.__ or __ UNITS NO INSULIN DOSE REQUIRED FOR MEALS/SNACKS UNDER __G OF CARBS OR EQUAL TO __.__ OR LESS	TIME __ :__ AM / PM LEFT ARM CGM / RIGHT ARM CGM / LEFT LEG CGM / RIGHT LEG CGM / LEFT/RIGHT STOMACH CGM KETONES NEGATIVE / TRACE / SMALL / MODERATE / LARGE
BEDTIME __ : __ PM	BLOOD SUGAR _____ UNITS ___ LEFT ARM CGM / RIGHT ARM CGM / LEFT LEG CGM / RIGHT LEG CGM / LEFT/RIGHT STOMACH CGM KETONES NEGATIVE / TRACE / SMALL / MODERATE / LARGE	HYDRATE 2AM BLOOD SUGAR _____ ADDITIONAL BLOOD SUGAR READINGS BS ___ at __ : __ AM/PM BS ___ at __ : __ AM/PM	NOTES MEDICINE

DATE: ______________________________ SUN MON TUES WED THUR FRI SAT

	MEALS AND SNACKS	CARB AND FOOD CALCULATIONS	SHOT DETAILS AND LOCATION
BREAKFAST	Total Carbohydrates : ___._ grams	Correction Dose: (BS - ___) / __ (___-___)/__ = (__/__) = ___.__ Carb Dose Calculation: (Meal Carbs / ___) (__._ /___) = ___.__ Correction Dose + Carb Dose Calculation: (__.__ + __.__) = __.__ OR __ UNITS Correction Dose / Dose Calculation / Rounded to nearest whole number	TIME __ : __ AM / PM LEFT ARM CGM / RIGHT ARM CGM / LEFT LEG CGM / RIGHT LEG CGM / LEFT/RIGHT STOMACH CGM KETONES NEGATIVE / TRACE / SMALL / MODERATE / LARGE
SNACK	Total Carbohydrates : ___._ grams	Carb Dose Calculation: (Meal Carbs / ___) (__._ /___) = ___.__ or __ UNITS NO INSULIN DOSE REQUIRED FOR MEALS/SNACKS UNDER __G OF CARBS OR EQUAL TO __.__ OR LESS	TIME __ : __ AM / PM LEFT ARM CGM / RIGHT ARM CGM / LEFT LEG CGM / RIGHT LEG CGM / LEFT/RIGHT STOMACH CGM KETONES NEGATIVE / TRACE / SMALL / MODERATE / LARGE
LUNCH	Total Carbohydrates : ___._ grams	Correction Dose: (BS - ___) / __ (___-___)/__ = (__/__) = ___.__ Carb Dose Calculation: (Meal Carbs / ___) (__._ /___) = ___.__ Correction Dose + Carb Dose Calculation: (__.__ + __.__) = __.__ OR __ UNITS Correction Dose / Dose Calculation / Rounded to nearest whole number	TIME __ : __ AM / PM LEFT ARM CGM / RIGHT ARM CGM / LEFT LEG CGM / RIGHT LEG CGM / LEFT/RIGHT STOMACH CGM KETONES NEGATIVE / TRACE / SMALL / MODERATE / LARGE
SNACK	Total Carbohydrates : ___._ grams	Carb Dose Calculation: (Meal Carbs / ___) (__._ /___) = ___.__ or __ UNITS NO INSULIN DOSE REQUIRED FOR MEALS/SNACKS UNDER __G OF CARBS OR EQUAL TO __.__ OR LESS	TIME __ : __ AM / PM LEFT ARM CGM / RIGHT ARM CGM / LEFT LEG CGM / RIGHT LEG CGM / LEFT/RIGHT STOMACH CGM KETONES NEGATIVE / TRACE / SMALL / MODERATE / LARGE
DINNER	Total Carbohydrates : ___._ grams	Correction Dose: (BS - ___) / __ (___-___)/__ = (__/__) = ___.__ Carb Dose Calculation: (Meal Carbs / ___) (__._ /___) = ___.__ Correction Dose + Carb Dose Calculation: (__.__ + __.__) = __.__ OR __ UNITS Correction Dose / Dose Calculation / Rounded to nearest whole number	TIME __ : __ AM / PM LEFT ARM CGM / RIGHT ARM CGM / LEFT LEG CGM / RIGHT LEG CGM / LEFT/RIGHT STOMACH CGM KETONES NEGATIVE / TRACE / SMALL / MODERATE / LARGE
SNACK	Total Carbohydrates : ___._ grams	Carb Dose Calculation: (Meal Carbs / ___) (__._ /___) = ___.__ or __ UNITS NO INSULIN DOSE REQUIRED FOR MEALS/SNACKS UNDER __G OF CARBS OR EQUAL TO __.__ OR LESS	TIME __ : __ AM / PM LEFT ARM CGM / RIGHT ARM CGM / LEFT LEG CGM / RIGHT LEG CGM / LEFT/RIGHT STOMACH CGM KETONES NEGATIVE / TRACE / SMALL / MODERATE / LARGE
BEDTIME __ : __ PM	BLOOD SUGAR ____ UNITS ___ LEFT ARM CGM / RIGHT ARM CGM / LEFT LEG CGM / RIGHT LEG CGM / LEFT/RIGHT STOMACH CGM KETONES NEGATIVE / TRACE / SMALL / MODERATE / LARGE	HYDRATE 2AM BLOOD SUGAR ____ ADDITIONAL BLOOD SUGAR READINGS BS ___ at __ : __ AM/PM BS ___ at __ : __ AM/PM	NOTES MEDICINE

DATE: ______________________ SUN MON TUES WED THUR FRI SAT

	MEALS AND SNACKS	CARB AND FOOD CALCULATIONS	SHOT DETAILS AND LOCATION
BREAKFAST	Total Carbohydrates : ___._ grams	Correction Dose: (BS - ___) / __ (___-___)/__ = (__/__) = ___.__ Carb Dose Calculation: (Meal Carbs / ___) (__._ /___) = ___.__ Correction Dose + Carb Dose Calculation: (_____ + _____) = __.__ OR __ UNITS Correction Dose Dose Calculation Rounded to nearest whole number	TIME __ : __ AM / PM LEFT ARM CGM | RIGHT ARM CGM | LEFT LEG CGM | RIGHT LEG CGM | LEFT/RIGHT STOMACH CGM KETONES NEGATIVE TRACE SMALL MODERATE LARGE
SNACK	Total Carbohydrates : ___._ grams	Carb Dose Calculation: (Meal Carbs / ___) (__._ /___) = ___.__ or __ UNITS NO INSULIN DOSE REQUIRED FOR MEALS/SNACKS UNDER __G OF CARBS OR EQUAL TO __.__ OR LESS	TIME __ : __ AM / PM LEFT ARM CGM | RIGHT ARM CGM | LEFT LEG CGM | RIGHT LEG CGM | LEFT/RIGHT STOMACH CGM KETONES NEGATIVE TRACE SMALL MODERATE LARGE
LUNCH	Total Carbohydrates : ___._ grams	Correction Dose: (BS - ___) / __ (___-___)/__ = (__/__) = ___.__ Carb Dose Calculation: (Meal Carbs / ___) (__._ /___) = ___.__ Correction Dose + Carb Dose Calculation: (_____ + _____) = __.__ OR __ UNITS Correction Dose Dose Calculation Rounded to nearest whole number	TIME __ : __ AM / PM LEFT ARM CGM | RIGHT ARM CGM | LEFT LEG CGM | RIGHT LEG CGM | LEFT/RIGHT STOMACH CGM KETONES NEGATIVE TRACE SMALL MODERATE LARGE
SNACK	Total Carbohydrates : ___._ grams	Carb Dose Calculation: (Meal Carbs / ___) (__._ /___) = ___.__ or __ UNITS NO INSULIN DOSE REQUIRED FOR MEALS/SNACKS UNDER __G OF CARBS OR EQUAL TO __.__ OR LESS	TIME __ : __ AM / PM LEFT ARM CGM | RIGHT ARM CGM | LEFT LEG CGM | RIGHT LEG CGM | LEFT/RIGHT STOMACH CGM KETONES NEGATIVE TRACE SMALL MODERATE LARGE
DINNER	Total Carbohydrates : ___._ grams	Correction Dose: (BS - ___) / __ (___-___)/__ = (__/__) = ___.__ Carb Dose Calculation: (Meal Carbs / ___) (__._ /___) = ___.__ Correction Dose + Carb Dose Calculation: (_____ + _____) = __.__ OR __ UNITS Correction Dose Dose Calculation Rounded to nearest whole number	TIME __ : __ AM / PM LEFT ARM CGM | RIGHT ARM CGM | LEFT LEG CGM | RIGHT LEG CGM | LEFT/RIGHT STOMACH CGM KETONES NEGATIVE TRACE SMALL MODERATE LARGE
SNACK	Total Carbohydrates : ___._ grams	Carb Dose Calculation: (Meal Carbs / ___) (__._ /___) = ___.__ or __ UNITS NO INSULIN DOSE REQUIRED FOR MEALS/SNACKS UNDER __G OF CARBS OR EQUAL TO __.__ OR LESS	TIME __ : __ AM / PM LEFT ARM CGM | RIGHT ARM CGM | LEFT LEG CGM | RIGHT LEG CGM | LEFT/RIGHT STOMACH CGM KETONES NEGATIVE TRACE SMALL MODERATE LARGE
BEDTIME __ : __ PM	BLOOD SUGAR ____ UNITS ___ LEFT ARM CGM | RIGHT ARM CGM | LEFT LEG CGM | RIGHT LEG CGM | LEFT/RIGHT STOMACH CGM KETONES NEGATIVE TRACE SMALL MODERATE LARGE	HYDRATE 2AM BLOOD SUGAR ____ ADDITIONAL BLOOD SUGAR READINGS BS ___ at __ : __ AM/PM BS ___ at __ : __ AM/PM	NOTES MEDICINE

DATE: ______________________ SUN MON TUES WED THUR FRI SAT

	MEALS AND SNACKS	CARB AND FOOD CALCULATIONS	SHOT DETAILS AND LOCATION
BREAKFAST	Total Carbohydrates : ___._ grams	Correction Dose: (BS - ___) / __ (___-___)/__ = (__/__) = ___.__ Carb Dose Calculation: (Meal Carbs / ___) (__._ /___) = ___.__ Correction Dose + Carb Dose Calculation: (__.__ + __.__) = __.__ OR __ UNITS Correction Dose / Dose Calculation / Rounded to nearest whole number	TIME __ : __ AM / PM LEFT ARM CGM / RIGHT ARM CGM / LEFT LEG CGM / RIGHT LEG CGM / LEFT/RIGHT STOMACH CGM KETONES NEGATIVE TRACE SMALL MODERATE LARGE
SNACK	Total Carbohydrates : ___._ grams	Carb Dose Calculation: (Meal Carbs / ___) (__._ /___) = ___.__ or __ UNITS NO INSULIN DOSE REQUIRED FOR MEALS/SNACKS UNDER __G OF CARBS OR EQUAL TO __.__ OR LESS	TIME __ : __ AM / PM LEFT ARM CGM / RIGHT ARM CGM / LEFT LEG CGM / RIGHT LEG CGM / LEFT/RIGHT STOMACH CGM KETONES NEGATIVE TRACE SMALL MODERATE LARGE
LUNCH	Total Carbohydrates : ___._ grams	Correction Dose: (BS - ___) / __ (___-___)/__ = (__/__) = ___.__ Carb Dose Calculation: (Meal Carbs / ___) (__._ /___) = ___.__ Correction Dose + Carb Dose Calculation: (__.__ + __.__) = __.__ OR __ UNITS Correction Dose / Dose Calculation / Rounded to nearest whole number	TIME __ : __ AM / PM LEFT ARM CGM / RIGHT ARM CGM / LEFT LEG CGM / RIGHT LEG CGM / LEFT/RIGHT STOMACH CGM KETONES NEGATIVE TRACE SMALL MODERATE LARGE
SNACK	Total Carbohydrates : ___._ grams	Carb Dose Calculation: (Meal Carbs / ___) (__._ /___) = ___.__ or __ UNITS NO INSULIN DOSE REQUIRED FOR MEALS/SNACKS UNDER __G OF CARBS OR EQUAL TO __.__ OR LESS	TIME __ : __ AM / PM LEFT ARM CGM / RIGHT ARM CGM / LEFT LEG CGM / RIGHT LEG CGM / LEFT/RIGHT STOMACH CGM KETONES NEGATIVE TRACE SMALL MODERATE LARGE
DINNER	Total Carbohydrates : ___._ grams	Correction Dose: (BS - ___) / __ (___-___)/__ = (__/__) = ___.__ Carb Dose Calculation: (Meal Carbs / ___) (__._ /___) = ___.__ Correction Dose + Carb Dose Calculation: (__.__ + __.__) = __.__ OR __ UNITS Correction Dose / Dose Calculation / Rounded to nearest whole number	TIME __ : __ AM / PM LEFT ARM CGM / RIGHT ARM CGM / LEFT LEG CGM / RIGHT LEG CGM / LEFT/RIGHT STOMACH CGM KETONES NEGATIVE TRACE SMALL MODERATE LARGE
SNACK	Total Carbohydrates : ___._ grams	Carb Dose Calculation: (Meal Carbs / ___) (__._ /___) = ___.__ or __ UNITS NO INSULIN DOSE REQUIRED FOR MEALS/SNACKS UNDER __G OF CARBS OR EQUAL TO __.__ OR LESS	TIME __ : __ AM / PM LEFT ARM CGM / RIGHT ARM CGM / LEFT LEG CGM / RIGHT LEG CGM / LEFT/RIGHT STOMACH CGM KETONES NEGATIVE TRACE SMALL MODERATE LARGE
BEDTIME __ : __ PM	BLOOD SUGAR ____ UNITS ___ LEFT ARM CGM / RIGHT ARM CGM / LEFT LEG CGM / RIGHT LEG CGM / LEFT/RIGHT STOMACH CGM KETONES NEGATIVE TRACE SMALL MODERATE LARGE	HYDRATE 2AM BLOOD SUGAR ____ ADDITIONAL BLOOD SUGAR READINGS BS ___ at __ : __ AM/PM BS ___ at __ : __ AM/PM	NOTES MEDICINE

NOTES

NOTES

NOTES

NOTES

NOTES

NOTES

NOTES

NOTES

NOTES

NOTES

Made in the USA
Monee, IL
02 November 2026

67381347R00063